Contents

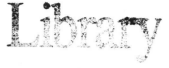

Forewords, iv

1 Introduction, 1

2 Osteoarthritis, Aetiology and Epidemiology, 4

3 Diagnosis and Differential Diagnosis of Osteoarthritis, 19

4 Examination of Joints, 33

5 Assessment of Osteoarthritis Including Hand Osteoarthritis, 55

6 Management Options—Education, Behavioural and Environmental, 66

7 Physical Therapy and Mechanical Interventions, 78

8 Pharmacological Treatment, 85

9 Surgical Options and Procedures, 98

10 Long-term Management and Referral, 115

11 Economic and Research Considerations, 121

Appendices

1 'GALS' Screening Examination, 127

2 WOMAC and Lequesne Scales, 128

3 Beighton Score, 130

4 Useful Addresses, 131

5 Further Reading, 133

6 Useful Websites, 136

Index, 138

Forewords

Foreword by Michael Doherty

Osteoarthritis (OA) is by far the commonest joint condition and a major cause of musculoskeletal pain and disability. Because of its strong association with ageing it will impose an even greater community burden as the 'greying' of the population continues.

Many factors favour the primacy of the general practice team in the management of OA. For example, the high prevalence of the condition; the generally benign outcome for many forms of OA; the importance of holistic clinical assessment for diagnosis and management; and the benefits of education, lifestyle modification and simple medications for the majority of patients.

This book is therefore welcome. Unlike other texts on OA this is the first to be written by GPs for a general practice audience. The 'front line' problem-based perspective clearly shines through, producing a very practical book of relevance to all UK Practitioners. The book, however, is not compromised by superficiality. Both authors have a special interest and expertise in musculoskeletal disease and each facet of OA is given comprehensive and up-to-date coverage.

I have no hesitation in commending this excellent book. Its reading should stimulate interest in this most common cause of pain and advance the standard of care received by millions of people in the UK.

Michael Doherty
Professor of Rheumatology
University of Nottingham Medical School
UK

Foreword by Peter Brooks

This book, written by GPs for GPs, is a useful addition to the growing number of rheumatological texts. Osteoarthritis is the most common musculo-skeletal disorder and should be managed primarily by GPs.

It is clearly written from a very practical perspective, highlighting 'Red Flag' conditions that need to be considered is an excellent way of alerting the reader to some of the pitfalls in differential diagnosis of joint pain. The authors emphasise the importance of history taking and examination and formulating a multi-faceted management plan. Investigation of osteoarthritis is appropriately de-emphasised but the chapters on therapy are comprehensive. Therapeutics in rheumatology is going through an exciting development particularly with the release of COX 2 specific inhibitors.

The discussion of surgical options is also excellent and emphasises the enormous benefits that can be gained from hip or knee replacement. Complementary therapies are also well covered, as these are commonly used by this group of patients. It is also nice to see a discussion of cost effectiveness and economics in a text such as this as these issues are not always appropriately considered by medical practitioners.

The emphasis in this book is on practical solutions coordinated by general practitioners in a primary care setting. This is highly appropriate for this disease and timely as we enter the Decade of Bone and Joint Disease—an initiative of Government agencies, professional and patient groups around the world to help focus the community on the burden of disease caused by OA and other musculoskeletal complaints.

Drs Hosie and Dickson are to be congratulated on their text, which will provide a good template for GPs and others managing OA in primary care.

Peter Brooks
Executive Dean (Health Sciences)
University of Queensland
Australia

Foreword by Kenneth Brandt

It has been reckoned that only 4% of patients with arthritis in the United States are ever seen by a rheumatologist. OA is unquestionably the province of the primary care physician.

It is important to recognise that impediments to the implementation of the good medical practices exist and are obstacles to the effective management of OA. For example, how, with a schedule requiring that they see a patient every 7 minutes or so, do primary care physicians appropriate the requisite time to transmit the practical information required by the patient to effect the behavioural changes needed for management of OA? Everything need not—and can not—be covered in a single office visit. Furthermore, because many patients with OA have significant comorbidities and are troubled, for example, by chronic cough, angina and diabetes, the gimpy knee often gets short shrift. This is a problem that can not be solved only by the caring and capable physician. It requires changes in the health care delivery system.

In addition, there is the unwarranted pessimism held by both physicians and patients—'there is nothing that can be done to help you.' Sadly, this is often the view even when the physician has a good understanding of pathophysiology and treatment options.

In crafting *Managing Osteoarthritis in Primary Care*, Gillian Hosie and John Dickson have provided a very useful guide for the generalist managing the patient with OA. While the Table of Contents may be no different from that of a textbook on OA written by a specialist in Rheumatology, the real value of this book lies in the authors' holistic approach to the patient with OA. Primary care physicians who take the time to read *Managing Osteoarthritis in Primary Care* are likely to refer to it repeatedly in dealing with their patients with OA.

For the patient with OA, the caregiver, the physician and the researcher in this area, the picture has never been brighter. With the use of better and safer drugs and non-medicinal measures, we are today able to treat OA symptoms more effectively and more safely than ever before. Furthermore, pharmacological agents and biologicals are being developed which, at least in animal models of OA, have shown the ability to prevent the development of structural damage in normal joints and/or slow the progression of damage in joints in which OA is already established.

This is, indeed, reason for optimism. It suggests that we may be on the threshold of a major change in our approach to management of OA and perhaps, even to pharmacological prevention of OA. Perhaps the correct perspective is provided by the words of Churchill, uttered, admittedly, in a very different context:

> *This is not the end. It is not even the beginning of the end. It is, perhaps, the end of the beginning.*
> W.S. Churchill, 1942 (the Battle of Alamein)

We hope that will be the case. However, even if they prove to be effective in humans, whether such drugs, which have been designated Disease-Modifying OA Drugs (DMOADs), will result in a decrease in joint pain, improvement in function, reduction in disability and in the need for costly joint replacement surgery remains to be determined.

How do we facilitate the physician's ability to transmit the best information to the patient? How do we get patients to do the things that informed health professionals recommend? 'Assembly line' visits are part of the problem, but by no means the entire problem. The authors allude to this issue in the section, 'Behaviour decisions of patients and doctors,' in Chapter 6. In enumerating the barriers which may keep the *person* with OA from consulting a GP—that is, from becoming a *patient* with OA—they provide useful insights. However, effecting behavioural changes in patients so that these issues are circumvented or eliminated is not easy. That, however, could serve as the topic for another book.

Kenneth D. Brandt, M.D.
Professor of Medicine and Head, Rheumatology Division
Indiana University School of Medicine
USA

CHAPTER 1

Introduction

Musculoskeletal problems are very common in primary care and represent around 15–20% of a GP's workload. Of these musculoskeletal problems many are due to osteoarthritis (OA) and the various problems it represents. For a long time there has been a negative approach to OA for the following reasons:
- It was thought to be an inevitable consequence of growing older.
- Management consisted only of pain control with analgesics and non-steroidal anti-inflammatory drugs (NSAIDs).
- NSAIDs were increasingly found to be causing major gastric side-effects, yet often doctors had little else to offer.
- Total joint replacements were undertaken late in the course of the disease when the patients were often too frail and unfit to obtain full benefit.
- Little research was undertaken into OA, as it was felt to be an unexciting and depressing condition.

Increasingly the situation is changing. While OA *is* more common in older age groups, not everyone will develop symptomatic OA as they age. Drug therapy is no longer the only management option but has become just one part of a much broader holistic approach. Much more research is being undertaken, looking at the epidemiology and progression of OA and potential ways of protecting cartilage from degradation, preventing OA in those people with known risk factors and in those with early disease, and also in preventing progression in those with established disease. With an increasing number of older people with justifiable expectations of living into active retirement, the demand for effective management of painful and disabling OA, both medical and surgical, will continue to rise and create a huge economic burden.

In this book all aspects of OA are considered from a community viewpoint to enable those of us working in primary care to manage our patients with OA effectively.

In Chapter 2 we look at the aetiology of OA and the risk factors, both modifiable and non-modifiable, for the development of the condition and its subsequent progression. The pathophysiology of OA is then described to show the relationship between pathology and clinical features.

In the next three chapters we discuss how, and by what criteria a diagnosis of OA is made in primary care. Chapter 3 considers the clinical manifestations of OA, together with differential diagnosis and the few cases where signs and symptoms would suggest some serious pathology requiring urgent attention ('Red Flags').

Chapter 4 describes the fundamentals of a hands-on examination of a patient with OA. Examination of joints is a skill which is often overlooked in both undergraduate and postgraduate training but which is essential in everyday primary care management.

Chapter 5 considers how to assess the individual patient in whom we have made a diagnosis of OA and considers pain, function and joint damage in both the short and long term. It also includes a practical guide to osteoarthritis of the hand, which includes useful knowledge for patient management in primary care.

Chapter 6 looks at OA in terms of general management and changing attitudes. Lack of mobility and pain can lead to problems at work, in the home and socially. Patients often have to make adjustments in their lifestyle, both with activities and in attitudes, to cope with problems caused by OA. This kind of behavioural change depends on education, both of patients and doctors, and the provision of educational material and opportunities to support both groups. It is important that patients, doctors, carers and the community are provided with the support and education to help OA sufferers, not merely cope but maintain a good quality of life. Long-term behavioural change depends on commitments by individuals, in terms of lifestyle change, and by the community in offering support for such change and in providing ways of aiding those disabled by OA in the community.

In Chapter 7 we discuss management by physical methods, encompassing physiotherapy and mechanical interventions, including aids, appliances and footwear.

It is important to look at management by physical and behavioural changes before pharmacological therapy as non-drug therapy is, at present, the most important aspect of long-term management of OA. Drug therapy also has an important part to play but this may be of less importance than was previously thought. Chapter 8 provides a comprehensive review of pharmacological management including topical and injection treatments, as well as analgesic and NSAID therapy.

The following chapter (Chapter 9) is devoted to surgery for OA and looks at possible surgical options available, including total joint replacement. Surgery has a very important part to play in the management of severe, painful and disabling OA, especially in the lower limb, but it is an option not always freely available and there may be a long waiting time: firstly for a surgical opinion and secondly for the operation itself.

If a patient with severe, painful, disabling OA is not suitable for operation or does not wish to consider this option, you may be faced with a difficult management problem. These patients look to us, as their primary care doctor, to provide continuing help and support. They may come to see us on a regular basis and in the face of this, we can feel useless and frustrated that we cannot solve their ongoing problems. In these instances, referral to another body or discipline may be helpful and Chapter 10 discusses the various options available.

In Chapter 11 we look briefly at economic and research considerations. OA with its management options of education, behavioural change, physical therapy, mechanical aids, drug therapy, surgical procedures and long-term care, costs the community a great deal of money. The individual who has OA, may incur extra costs for such things as transport and help in the home. Other health costs may also arise which may be difficult to quantify, such as loss of social life, social isolation and depression.

The future in OA management looks brighter now than it has ever done. We have greater understanding of some of the reasons for the development and progression of OA and, hopefully, these will give us some guidance in applying prevention. New drugs are being developed, some to provide better symptomatic relief, with fewer side-effects, and others to prevent cartilage breakdown and, therefore, to act as disease-modifying agents.

Much of the management of OA can be undertaken very effectively in primary care and we hope that this book will provide the primary care team with a practical and comprehensive guide to the diagnosis and management of OA in the community.

CHAPTER 2

Osteoarthritis, Aetiology and Epidemiology

Osteoarthritis (OA) is a condition which has affected mankind for many thousands of years. It has been found in skeletal remains, some dating as far back as Neolithic times. OA is not confined to the human species and causes many problems in domestic animals, especially in dogs and horses. There is a hypothesis, though no direct evidence, that the joints most affected by the osteoarthritic process are those which have most recently had a change of use as a result of evolution, for example the hip joint, as humans have gradually developed over thousands of years from a quadruped to a biped. Similar evolutionary changes have occurred at the base of the thumb, as the hand has adapted to improve grip with an opposing thumb.

OA is a very common condition and is probably the single biggest cause of disability due to the locomotor system. The definition of OA is difficult and there is considerable controversy as to whether it can be diagnosed on purely clinical grounds or whether diagnosis requires radiological confirmation. There is often poor correlation between clinical symptoms and X-ray changes. Some patients may have quite severe radiological changes, with very little in the way of symptoms, while others have severe symptoms with only minor radiological changes.

OA is thought to be a common end-stage product of joint failure resulting from a number of different influences or diseases acting on the joint. All joints can be affected by OA but by far the most common joints affected are knees, distal interphalangeal joints, base of thumb, hips and facet joints in the spine. OA is more common in women in all joints, except the hip, where the condition is equally prevalent between males and females.

Classification of osteoarthritis

For many years doctors have tried to classify OA, in terms of the following.
- Number of joints involved, e.g. monoarticular, polyarticular.
- Aetiology:
  1 primary—no obvious cause;
  2 secondary—past history of congenital abnormality or trauma.

- Clinical and radiographic picture, e.g. inflammatory, erosive, crystal deposition, and so on.

However, no perfect classification system yet exists.

There are a number of common clinical patterns of osteoarthritis as shown in Fig. 2.1 One of the most common is that of a middle-aged to elderly woman with OA of the knee and hand. Single joint OA often occurs in men. In younger men this is particularly common at the hip and may be related to dysplasia, while middle-aged men present more commonly with OA of one knee. Usually these patients have a past history of some major traumatic event affecting the joint. In elderly patients, most commonly in women, a severe form of OA may develop affecting many different joints particularly shoulders, knees and hips. These patients can suffer considerable pain and develop large effusions in the joints, often containing apatite crystals. This condition can cause bony destruction around the joint, as well as soft tissue damage and cartilage loss. When it occurs in the shoulder, it is called Milwaukee shoulder.

However, a large number of patients presenting with OA do not fit neatly into one of these clinical patterns. Some older patients may present for the first time with isolated hip or hand OA, many present with knee OA with no specific past history of trauma and often the knee problem is bilateral.

How and why do people develop osteoarthritis?

There are some recognized risk factors for the development of OA in particular joints, but like many medical conditions, having the risk factors does not necessarily lead to the development of OA. Conversely, many people with no obvious risk factors develop the condition. In certain individuals who seem to have a genetic predisposition to OA, exacerbating factors, such as abnormal loading applied to the joint, may cause the development of OA. Some of these factors are listed in Tables 2.1 and 2.2 and are discussed in the following paragraphs.

Table 2.1 General risk factors.

Genetic susceptibility
Obesity
Female sex
Increasing age
Menopausal oestrogen loss
Poor nutritional status

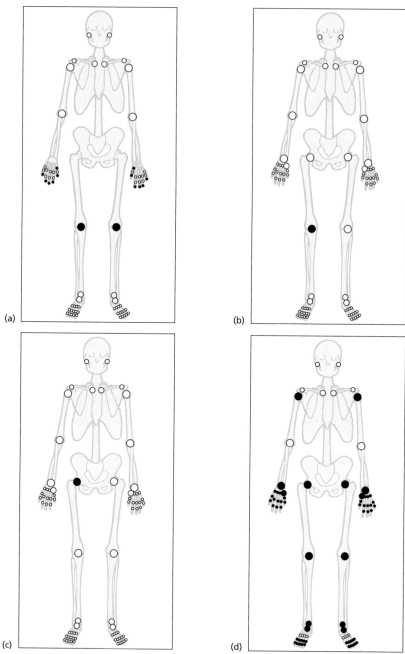

Fig. 2.1 Common clinical patterns in OA. (a) Middle-aged female with OA of knees and hands. (b) Middle-aged man with OA of one knee often due to previous trauma. (c) Young man with OA of one joint, usually hip. May be related to dysplasia, may have genetic collagen abnormalities. (d) Elderly female with severe OA affecting many joints but especially shoulders, hips and knees. Joints often show large effusions containing apatite crystals. This condition may cause bony destruction around the joint, together with soft tissue damage and cartilage loss. When it occurs in the shoulder it is called Milwaukee shoulder. (Arms internally rotated so palms face posteriorly.) From [12] with permission.

Table 2.2 Specific risk factors—abnormal loading.	Trauma
	    fracture
	    ligament damage
	    meniscal tears
	Dysplasia
	Childhood hip problems
	    Perthes' disease
	    dislocation of hip
	    slipped femoral epiphysis
	Hip pathology
	Unequal leg length
	Hypermobility
	Occupations involving bending and carrying

General risk factors

Genetic susceptibility

For an individual the risk of developing OA is likely to be a multifactorial mix of:
- Individual constitutional susceptibility;
- Local mechanical risk factors.

It has been known for over 50 years that there is a strong genetic influence on the development of nodal hand OA, particularly in women (Fig. 2.2). Although there are isolated reports of familial OA being associated with mutations in collagen genes, these have been from patients with atypical or premature disease.

Evidence for a genetic contribution to 'common OA' in the community has only recently been reported [1]. This evidence suggests that there is a strong genetic influence on the development of OA at the knee, hip, and spine as well as the hand. Although the precise genes are not yet known, the immediate clinical relevance is the identification of a positive family history (in parents or siblings) as a very strong risk factor.

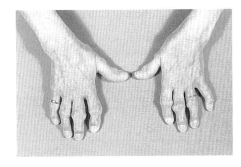

Fig. 2.2 Heberden's nodes of the DIP and Bouchard's nodes of the PIP joints. With permission from Professor R. Sturrock.

The relation of osteoarthritis and obesity

The long-term Framingham study in the USA and associated studies [2–5] have provided much valuable information about the association of knee OA and obesity. The results suggest that obesity predisposes to the development of OA in later life. It may be that the extra mechanical loading of obesity over many years causes the development of knee OA. More women than men have knee OA and more women suffer from obesity but the relationship between these two factors may not be direct.

Obesity appears to affect both the risk of developing OA and the clinical course of established OA. Weight loss of 5 kg (11 lb) in women with a body mass index of 25 or more, led to a 50% reduction in the risk of developing symptomatic knee OA [5] and a clinical trial looking at weight loss treatment showed a considerable correlation between the amount of weight loss and symptomatic improvement in patients with established knee OA [4].

The association of hip OA and obesity is less clear, although there is increasing evidence that obesity leads to a high risk of developing bilateral radiographic hip OA [6] and symptomatic hip OA [7,8].

There are two possible mechanisms for the association of obesity and OA.
- Extra mechanical loading, causing cartilage breakdown.
- Excess fatty tissue may produce abnormal hormone levels, which may affect bone and cartilage, although to date such hormones have not been identified.

The association of hand OA with obesity would suggest that mechanical forces are not the sole cause and in most cases of OA, both mechanisms probably work together.

Female sex and menopausal oestrogen loss

Below the age of 50, men have a higher prevalence of OA but after the age of 50, women have a higher prevalence (Fig. 2.3) and this is probably related to menopausal oestrogen loss. Many women develop OA around or shortly after the menopause and so a hormonal basis for the aetiology has been postulated. Recent research has shown the presence of oestrogen receptors on the surface of osteoblasts and further work is on-going in this field. Hormone replacement therapy (HRT) as well as helping some symptoms of OA, possibly by increasing general well-being and encouraging activity, has now been shown to reduce the risk of development of OA of hip and knee.

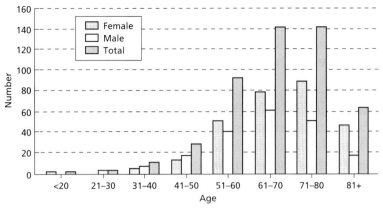

Fig. 2.3 The age/sex distribution of samples of OA patients. Data from questionnaires sent to OA patients in two UK practices. From J. Dickson and G. Hosie, unpublished data.

OA appears to be negatively associated with osteoporosis, especially at the hip joint, and patients who have hip OA are much less likely to sustain a fractured neck of femur. Increasing levels of circulating oestrogen with HRT may help to prevent both osteoporosis and OA.

Other pathologies within joints, such as septic arthritis or avascular necrosis, and childhood hip problems, such as congenital dislocation of the hip, Perthes' disease and slipped femoral epiphysis, may lead to the later development of OA, as may hypermobility and unequal leg length.

Increasing age

OA usually occurs in patients aged over 50. If OA develops earlier, in one single joint, this usually indicates some major alteration in the biomechanics of the joint, probably due to some form of previous trauma. The association of OA with increasing age is thought to be due to a number of factors as follows.

• A decrease in the responsiveness of repair mechanisms.

• A decrease in neuromuscular function, resulting in loss of protection to the joint.

• An increase in laxity of the ligaments around the joint, resulting in greater likelihood of injury.

Rarely OA develops in several joints before the age of 50. In this instance a systemic cause should be considered, such as acromegaly, haemachromatosis, ochronosis or possibly a genetic type 2 collagen abnormality.

This may be an attempt by the joint to increase the area available for articulation or possibly to help joint stability. Changes also occur in the bone surrounding the joint, with the development of areas of sclerosis and bone cysts. Sclerosis occurs as new bone forms to strengthen the existing bony trabecular structure. Bone cysts occur in areas where the articular cartilage is absent and form as a result of raised intra-articular pressure, which is then transmitted into the marrow of the surrounding bone. These cysts may continue to expand until the pressure is equalized. These abnormal changes are shown in Fig. 2.5 which shows a normal joint for comparison.

While the changes of regeneration are occurring, debris, consisting of the degradation products from cartilage, together with material such as bone hydroxyapatite crystal, is deposited in the joint space. This may lead to an inflammatory-type response, both pathologically and clinically, with the development of patchy areas of synovitis and increased viscosity of the synovial fluid. This inflammatory response may trigger further tissue destruction; eventually leading to effusion within the joint causing raised intra-articular pressure, with subsequent stretching and eventual thickening of the joint capsule.

Synovial fluid plays a role in the pathophysiology of OA, although this role has not been fully defined. Synovial fluid is not just a simple fluid or oil, it has a biological role and acts as a transport medium for all nutrients and, together with the synovial membrane, may have hormonal and messenger functions. Its major constituent is a hyaluronan. This is a polymerized glycosaminoglycan (previously called a mucopolysaccharide). In a normal joint, hyaluronan has a high molecular weight. These molecules give synovial fluid some of its biological properties so that the fluid is able to act as a shock absorber and as a lubricant. It has also been suggested that the larger molecules 'protect' the nociceptors (pain-mediating receptors) in joints.

In an OA joint, synovial fluid has hyaluronan of a lower molecular weight. It is unclear what part this lower molecular weight hyaluronan plays in the OA process, whether it is the result of the OA process, whether it is compensatory or even whether it is the initial change instigating the whole pathophysiological process.

Clinical features

Pain

The clinical features of OA are a reflection of the pathological changes taking place within the joint. Pain is the main symptom of OA. The pain

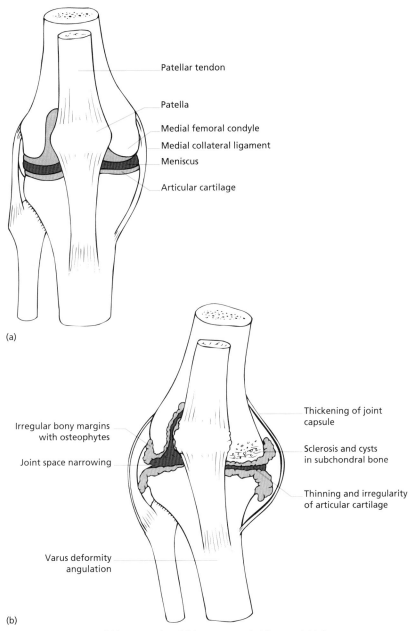

Patellar tendon

Patella
Medial femoral condyle
Medial collateral ligament
Meniscus

Articular cartilage

(a)

Thickening of joint capsule

Irregular bony margins with osteophytes

Joint space narrowing

Sclerosis and cysts in subchondral bone

Thinning and irregularity of articular cartilage

Varus deformity angulation

(b)

Fig. 2.5 Comparison of (a) a normal and (b) an osteoarthritic synovial joint.

is related to the use of the joint, while using the joint or immediately after use. This pain is often difficult to describe and may be a deep dull ache or a sharp severe pain. A number of different pathological processes may give rise to the pain felt in an OA joint as illustrated in Fig. 2.6.

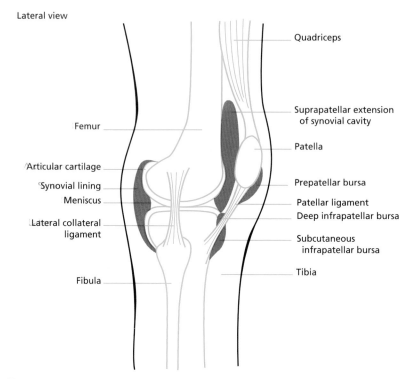

Lateral view

Quadriceps

Suprapatellar extension of synovial cavity

Femur

Patella

Articular cartilage

Prepatellar bursa

Synovial lining

Meniscus

Patellar ligament
Deep infrapatellar bursa

Lateral collateral ligament

Subcutaneous infrapatellar bursa

Fibula

Tibia

Fig. 2.6 Functional anatomy and causes of pain in and around the knee. From [13] with permission.

These processes include the following.
- Increased intracapsular pressure.
- Increased pressure in surrounding bone.
- Inflammation of the synovium.
- Periarticular problems, such as bursitis or enthesopathies.
- Alteration in muscle function around the joint.
- Periosteal changes.
- Abnormal pressure on the capsule and ligaments.

Stiffness

Pain is often accompanied by a degree of stiffness, which wears off fairly rapidly as the joint is used. It is most marked after a spell of immobility, such as lying in bed or sitting, and is often described as 'gelling'. The pathological cause of the stiffness in OA is not fully understood. It may be due to thickening of the capsule and alteration in the other periarticular structures or may relate to a degree of synovitis or fluid accumulation.

Functional impairment

Often in OA there is a decrease in the range of movement of the joint, probably due to bony changes, together with thickening of the capsule, preventing a full range of movement. Patients sometimes complain of a feeling that the joint is giving way and this may be due to weakness and impaired function of the muscles surrounding the joint.

Crepitus

Coarse crepitus is a common feature in an OA joint. This is felt (and sometimes heard) on movement of the joint and is thought to be due to irregularities in the joint surface with osteophytes and chondrocytes at the joint edges, preventing the usual smooth movement of the joint.

Bony changes

The growth of osteophytes at the joint margins causes bony swellings around the joint and clinically this leads to enlargement of the joint, with firm, occasionally tender swelling and changes in the appearance of the joint, often described as 'squaring' (Fig. 2.7).

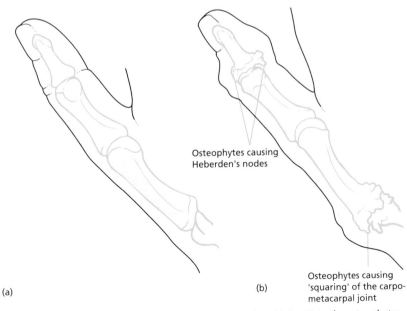

Osteophytes causing Heberden's nodes

Osteophytes causing 'squaring' of the carpo-metacarpal joint

(a)   (b)

Fig. 2.7 (a) A normal hand joint and (b) an osteoarthritic hand joint. Note the osteophytes and the subsequent deformity of contour or 'squaring' at the CMC joint.

Soft tissue swelling

Soft tissue swelling in an OA joint may be due to synovitis and there may be an effusion present. Effusions are usually cool but may be warm during an inflammatory flare. Many OA joints will have a small effusion present, probably reflecting a mild degree of chronic synovitis. Soft tissue swelling around the joint may also involve periarticular structures, such as bursae.

Joint destruction

In severe, long-standing OA, obvious deformity of the joints can occur due to destruction of the cartilage and underlying bone and surrounding soft tissue. When this occurs in the medial compartment of the knee, it leads to a typical varus angulation (Fig. 2.8a). Inflammatory arthritis, e.g. rheumatoid arthritis, typically causes valgus deformity (Fig. 2.8b).

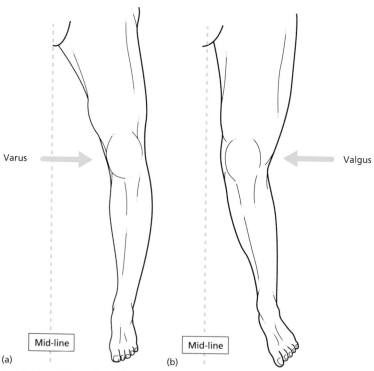

Fig. 2.8 OA tends to produce (a) varus, in contrast to rheumatoid arthritis, which produces (b) valgus deformity of the knee.

Prognosis

OA usually develops slowly but there may be periods of more rapid progression before the joint stabilizes again. Joints can often show clinical, and occasionally radiographic, improvement. Most patients who develop symptomatic OA suffer only intermittent problems of pain and reduced functional capacity, and can often relate symptomatic flares to a specific and perhaps unaccustomed mechanical stress. Some 40–50% of patients with OA, however, suffer on-going pain on a daily basis and require a variety of interventions as management, while around 10% of patients suffer extreme pain from their OA and become increasingly incapacitated by their condition, eventually developing end-stage disease.

Summary points

- Focal loss of cartilage in the joint is accompanied by hypertrophic reaction in the subchondral bone and the margin of the joint.
- X-ray changes include joint space narrowing, subchondral sclerosis and cyst formation and marginal osteophytosis.
- OA is very common and age related, and most commonly affects knees, hips, hands and facet joints of spine.
- Clinical features include age-related joint pain, gelling of joints after inactivity and decreased range of joint movement.
- X-ray changes often correlate poorly with clinical symptoms.
- Most people who develop OA will not be greatly incapacitated.
- OA is rarely progressive and stabilizes in most people.

References

1 MacGregor AJ. The genetics of Osteoarthritis. *ARC Topical Review* 1999; 16.
2 Felson DT, Zhang Y, Hannan MT *et al*. Risk factors for incident radiographic knee osteoarthritis in the elderly. *Arthritis Rheum* 1997; 40: 728–33.
3 Dougados M, Gueguen A, Nguyen M *et al*. Longitudinal radiologic evaluation of osteoarthritis of the knee. *J Rheumatol* 1992; 19: 378–83.
4 Williams RA, Foulsham BM. Weight reduction in osteoarthritis using phentermine. *Practitioner* 1981; 225: 231–2.
5 Felson DT, Zhang Y, Anthony JM, Naimark A, Anderson JJ. Weight loss reduces the risk for symptomatic knee osteoarthritis in women. *Ann Intern Med* 1992; 116: 535–9.

6   Nevitt NC, Lane NE, Scott JC, Genant HK, Hochberg MC. Relationship of hip osteoarthritis to obesity and bone mineral density in older American women: preliminary results from the Study of Osteoporotic Fractures. *Acta Orthop Scand* 1993; 64 (Suppl.): 2–5.

7   Roach KE, Persky V, Miles T, Budiman-Mak E. Biochemical aspects of occupation and osteoarthritis of the hip: a case–control study. *J Rheumatol* 1994; 21: 2334–40.

8   Kraus JF, D'Ambrosia RD, Smith EG *et al.* An epidemiological study of severe osteoarthritis. *Orthopedics* 1978; 1: 37–42.

9   Kirkeskov Jensen L, Eenberg W. Occupation as a risk factor for knee disorders. *Scand J Work Environ Health* 1996; 22: 165–75.

10 Hannan MT, Naimark A, Berkeley J, Gordon G, Wilson PWF, Anderson J. Occupational physical demands, knee bending, and knee osteoarthritis: results from the Framingham Study. *J Rheumatol* 1991; 18: 1587–92.

11 Croft P, Coggan D, Cruddas M, Cooper C. Osteoarthritis of the hip: an occupational disease in farmers. *BMJ* 1992; 304: 1269–72.

12 *Diploma in Primary Care Rheumatology by Distance Learning.* University of Bath and Primary Care Rheumatology Society.

13 Dieppe P, Kerwin J, Cooper C & McGill N. *Arthritis and Rheumatism in Practice.* London: Gower.

CHAPTER 3

Diagnosis and Differential Diagnosis of Osteoarthritis

Classical signs of osteoarthritis

In primary care, pattern recognition is extremely important—it helps us to make a diagnosis. When the pattern is not a good match to what we would expect, we should be considering alternative diagnoses. We will consider the 'model' patterns of osteoarthritis (OA) after we have discussed 'Red Flags'.

Knee OA is the commonest joint presenting with OA in primary care and, unless stated, the knee joint will be discussed as the model joint. It is important to remember that OA can affect any synovial joint. Common joints to be affected are shown in Table 3.1 and Fig. 3.1.

There are no diagnostic tests, either laboratory or X-ray, which will conclusively confirm or exclude OA. It is essentially a clinical diagnosis. Investigation may occasionally be useful in helping with a differential diagnosis, e.g. polymyalgia, where an erythrocyte sedimentation rate (ESR) is worth checking.

The concept of 'Red Flags' has become widely used since the worldwide implementation of back pain guidelines [1]. The concept is useful here too.

'Red Flags' for joint pain

When patients present with a joint problem, it is essential to exclude 'Red Flags'. There are three causes of joint pain which demand urgent attention and usually urgent patient referral.

Table 3.1 Synovial joints commonly affected by osteoarthritis.

Knees
Hips
Distal phalangeal joints of the hands
Interphalangeal joints of the hands
Sterno- and acromioclavicular joints
First carpometacarpal joints of the thumbs
First metatarsophalangeal joints of the foot
Facet joints of the spine

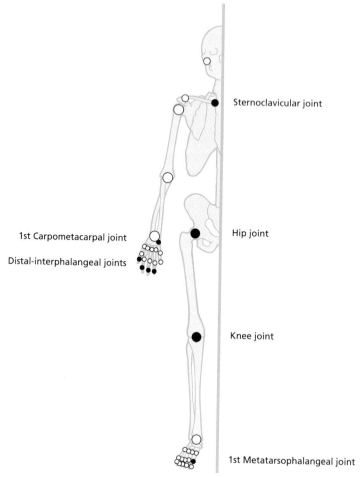

Fig. 3.1 Common synovial joints affected by OA.

- Septic arthritis.
- Bony fracture around the joint.
- Major ligamentous injury.

Features which should raise suspicion

If a patient presents with a hot swollen joint, septic arthritis must be excluded. The other cause would be acute gout. A severely inflamed joint from inflammatory arthritis is not 'this hot' unless it is septic. Figure 3.2 shows a septic shoulder.

Beware of patients who are on oral steroids or who have been given a steroid injection into the joint. In these patients the systemic signs of

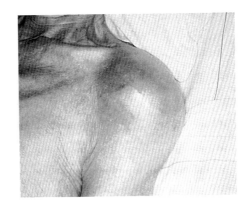

Fig. 3.2 Septic shoulder.

infection may be less severe, for example the joint may be red, swollen and cool, i.e. not hot. If in doubt it is best to refer or admit the patient; certainly ask for advice.

Pain in a joint following severe trauma could be due to a fracture or a ligament rupture. Suspect a serious cause of joint pain in a weight-bearing joint (e.g. knee) if the patient cannot weight bear or move the joint.

Cancer pain

This pain is usually severe, constant and progressive, becoming very severe and it is rarely relieved by the common analgesics. It is a rare cause of single joint pain in an adult.

Clinical pattern for osteoarthritis of the knee

- The person is likely to be aged over 50.
- The person has use-related knee pain. This can be on walking or standing.
- The joint has a tendency to stiffen after prolonged inactivity, so requires loosening up when activity is restarted (hence the phrase from the patient 'It will be alright once I get going again').
- There is creaking (crepitus) of the joint as it is moved—felt by a hand on the joint, or in some instances this crepitus may be heard.
- The knee joint becomes harder, or firmer and more square. Sometimes there is a mild deformity or a change in the movement of the joint.

Some of these features will be appropriate to other joints with OA. For example, the acromio- and sternoclavicular joints and the first metatarsophalangeal joints may have crepitus when moved. Most OA joints will become firmer, larger and appear squarer than their normal comparator joints, e.g. distal interphalangeal joints with Heberden's nodes.

3

It is always worth comparing joints on both sides, but beware as both sides may be abnormal, e.g. knees, though often one is worse than the other (usually the dominant or lead leg). Few patients presenting with possible OA, are under 50 years old unless there has been a secondary provoking factor such as a previous fracture or a sports injury affecting tendons or cartilage. In this context, do not forget childhood problems such as slipped femoral epiphysis or previous Perthes' disease.

Presenting signs and symptoms

We can now move on to the patient's presenting problems which are listed in Table 3.2. Patients commonly present complaining of pain in or around a joint. Also, loss of function, such as loss of mobility or problems with a hobby (holding a golf club or problems while gardening) may initiate an appointment. A few patients are more worried about the appearance of lumps and bumps, especially on their hands or knees, or even a knee angulation and it is this, rather than the pain, that makes patients present. The other signs and presenting symptoms are listed in Table 3.2. Patients may present with any one or any combination of symptoms.

Features of the pain

Patients describe pain variably as:
- aching in and around the knee;
- persistent pain in and around the knee;
- intermittent acute, stabbing pain.

In early disease, pain is often just an ache that can become worse on standing or on the initiation of an attempt to walk: it may be present during a viral infection such as one involving the upper respiratory tract.

Pain
Crepitus
Stiffness or gelling
Insecurity of the knees
Bony swelling or deformity (e.g. varus angulation)
Loss of joint movement (loss of mobility), e.g. limp caused by hip disease
Joint effusion
Joint tenderness on palpation

Table 3.2 Common presenting signs and symptoms of OA.

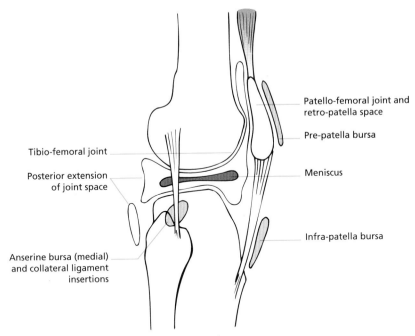

Patello-femoral joint and
retro-patella space

Pre-patella bursa

Tibio-femoral joint

Meniscus

Posterior extension
of joint space

Infra-patella bursa

Anserine bursa (medial)
and collateral ligament
insertions

Fig. 3.3 Potential sites for knee pain. From [2] with permission.

Remember that the pain often persists for a variable amount of time after stopping activity. Later, if the disease progresses, pain may be present at rest and may even waken the patient from sleep. Pain may be worse in cold or damp weather. Emotional factors and tiredness may have an affect on pain perception and intensity. The intensity of the pain may be so great that it limits or restricts mobility.

Common causes of knee pain

If a patient is aged 45 or more, OA is the most likely cause of the pain—though this is not always the case. To differentiate this condition, and to help with management strategies, we will discuss various classifications of knee pain according to site (Fig. 3.3), age and sex, and discuss the conditions that may be confused with OA (Table 3.3).

Site of the pain

Joint pain (articular pain)

Pain may arise from structures in the joint, i.e. from menisci or the cruciate ligaments. Pain from inflammation of the synovial membrane occurs in OA, though to a lesser extent compared to rheumatoid arthritis. In OA there may be bone pain as well.

Periarticular pain

Periarticular pain arises from structures around the joint. There may be ligament strains or tears (e.g. the collateral ligaments), inflammation of a bursa causing a bursitis, or pain at insertion of a tendon (enthesopathy). Pain from muscles adjacent to a joint may also occur.

Pain referred to the knee

Hip pain may be referred to the knee; in fact hip disease is a common cause of knee pain. This applies to patients of any age. The pain is usually anterior and above the knee but it may feel as if it comes from inside the knee joint. Remember to examine the hip and back especially if there is no quadriceps wasting. Referred pain can often be relieved, or partially relieved, by rubbing. It is unclear why this is so. It may be that rubbing acts as a counterirritant. The spine may also refer pain to the knee but this is less common.

Common causes of knee pain at different ages

We have already discussed pattern recognition as an aid to diagnosis and we can take this further, again using the knee as an example. The age and sex of the patient will indicate the most likely cause of the knee pain. Remember to use the three sources of pain (articular, periarticular and referred). Examples are shown in Table 3.3.

Common painful conditions that may confuse the clinical picture

Consider an alternative diagnosis in the following circumstances.
- The patient is under 45 years old.
- If the patient is ill or febrile then the patient is more likely to have sepsis, gout or a viral arthralgia.
- There is major loss of function, morning stiffness and inflammation; this suggests rheumatoid arthritis.
- Less commonly affected joints are involved, e.g. wrist, elbow, shoulder and ankle.

Table 3.3 Knee pain and age.

Age	Causes Articular	Periarticular	Referred
Children	Osteochondritis dissecans (M > F)	Bursitis	Hip disease
	Meniscal lesions	Osgood–Schlatter disease	
	Juvenile chronic arthritis		
	Anterior knee pain syndrome (F > M)		
Young adults	Meniscal injury	Fractures	Hip disease
	Cruciate ligament injury	Collateral ligament injuries	
	Inflammatory arthritis (reactive M > F, rheumatoid arthritis F > M)	Bursitis	
	Anterior knee pain syndrome (e.g. chondromalacia patellae F > M)		
Adults >45	Osteoarthritis (F > M)	Bursitis	Hip disease
	Fractures		
	Meniscal injury		
	Rarer causes, e.g. inflammatory arthritis (gout, rheumatoid arthritis, psoriatic arthritis, pseudogout)		

Ligamentous injury/periarticular areas

Who: Any age or sex

Pain: Bursitis or injury can mimic the pain of OA from an adjoining joint

What may confuse?
- An elderly person who has recently fallen without fracturing may complain of hip pain—this may be a trochanteric bursitis
- Patients with known hip or knee arthritis may walk 'abnormally' and develop a trochanteric or anserine bursitis
- Meniscal and other knee problems may develop in an OA knee. The rough and tumble of life may have caused an injury and not a flare of OA (see Chapter 4)

Fibromyalgia

Who: Age 40 to 50   F > M

Pain: Axial (neck and back, may be all over)
Tender points often periarticular (Fig. 3.4), e.g. medial fat pad of knee
Subjective swelling of hands
Morning stiffness
Non-restorative sleep/fatiguability and headaches

What may confuse?

Patients who are under 50 with pain all over are more likely to
have fibromyalgia. Look for associated syndromes. Pain from
generalized OA is more likely in older patients who may be
depressed

Associated syndromes:

Irritable bowel/dysmenorrhoea, menorrhagia and headaches

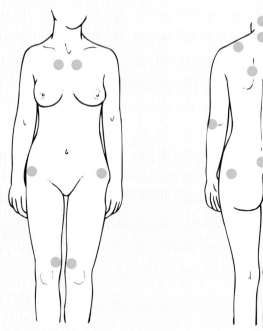

Fig. 3.4 Common tender areas in fibromyalgia.

Gout

Who: Male any age
Female postmenopausal

Pain: *Acute attack*: pain so severe that it is unlikely to be confused with OA
more chronic attack: less severe pain may occur in patients only partially controlled on allopurinol

What may confuse?
A chronic attack can be difficult to differentiate from OA—be alert if your patient is taking allopurinol, or is on thiazides or low dose aspirin or has changed diet

Features of chronic attacks
- Commonly affects proximal interphalangeal joints and distal joint nodes
- May affect only one joint
- May be Heberden's nodes and other features of OA
- Thiazide introduced to control blood pressure may produce loss of gout control and painful proximal interphalangeal joints or 'hot Heberden's nodes' (distal interphalangeal joints)

Features of acute attacks
Commonly affects first metatarsophalangeal joint
May involve heel, ankle and knee. Lower limb involvement more common than the upper limb. Ninety per cent of attacks affect only one joint

Investigations
- Uric acid level usually raised though may be lower during acute attack. Level may not be low enough to stop chronic attacks
- Polarization microscopy for crystals

Treatment
- If on thiazides—discontinue
- Treat inflammation with non-steroidal anti-inflammatory drug (NSAID) or, if contraindicated, Colchicine
- Consider allopurinol if recurrent attacks
- Consider asking for advice

3

Rheumatoid arthritis

Who: Any age, either sex. Usually a *misdiagnosis* rather than a differential one

Features:
- Morning stiffness and fatigue
- Pattern of joint involvement favours metacarpal, proximal interphalangeal and wrists
- Synovial swelling is soft (unlike the hard bony swelling of OA)
- Function is affected significantly. Even in early disease joints move slowly
- Joint pain is significant both on movement and on palpation

What may confuse?
Patients who present with local pain, redness and swelling especially of the distal interphalangeal joints. Acute signs settle over a few weeks or months with little, if any, loss of function and no systemic symptoms. This is OA.

Investigations: None diagnostic as both OA and RA at this early stage are clinical diagnoses. Look for normochromic and normocytic anaemia in RA. Hypochromic anaemia is due to iron loss (consider NSAID consumption or menorrhagia).

Polymyalgia rheumatica (PMR)

Cause: Unknown, may follow flu-like illness

Who: Rare under 55 years

Features:
- Diffuse muscle pain over shoulder or pelvic girdles, often with tenderness
- Difficulty in turning over in bed and stiffness especially after resting

Investigation: A high erythrocyte sedimentation rate (ESR)

What may confuse?
PMR superimposed on joints with mild to moderate OA

Treatment: Use moderate doses of steroids (15 mg). Usually good response in 3 days. Question your diagnosis if not responding to this dose in 1 week

Pseudogout

Cause: Pyrophosphate crystals released from articular cartilage

Who: Males and especially females aged 70 or more

Pain: Acute attack of inflammatory arthritis

Investigations
- By polarizing microscopy for crystals
- Synovial fluid culture to exclude sepsis
- Line of chondrocalcinosis on X-ray

What may confuse?
- Patient with a flare of 'osteoarthritis' in a somewhat atypical joint(s) pattern (wrists, shoulders or knee). Patient may wake up with stiff, warm, painful wrist which settles quickly if given NSAID. Next attack a few months later affects another joint
- Other patterns resemble acute gout or acute sepsis or a less severe attack of inflammatory arthritis
- The OA flare is usually less severe than an attack of pseudogout. Pseudogout often attacks a range of joints which respond to treatment quicker than an OA flare
- Think of the diagnosis in a patient who is female and over 70 with a painful, stiff joint. If a knee joint, there is invariably valgus angulation (knock knees—see Fig. 2.8)

Treatment: Less severe attacks respond well to NSAID. Others may need specialist advice for aspiration and exclusion of sepsis (which may coexist)

Psychological effects

Who: Patients with controlled mild to moderate OA of one or more joints

Pain: Emotional effects and stressful situations may disrupt this balance and patients begin to find the pain intolerable

What may confuse?
It is easy to miss the anxiety/depression element and concentrate on the 'OA pain' instead of counselling and appropriate medications

Other symptoms of osteoarthritis

Stiffness or 'gelling' of the joint

Sometimes a patient's presenting complaint may be that their knee (or other joint) gets 'stuck' after resting and it takes a little while (minutes) to get going again. Very often these patients are more worried about the joint stopping working completely than the ache or pain in the joint. Stiffness may be the first sign of OA or an OA flare. Certainly the painful stiffness may engender a tremendous amount of anxiety and even fear of becoming disabled—this may lead to mild depression.

Stiffness usually wears off after a few minutes' activity although some patients have morning stiffness wearing off after 30 min or so. Patients with synovitis and inflammatory arthritis, usually have morning stiffness for much longer. Naturally, if the OA is primarily affecting the hands, then there may be cause for confusion (see Chapter 5, Assessment of hand osteoarthritis). As already stated, loss of function is much greater in inflammatory arthritis.

Insecurity of the knee

Commonly, patients complain of, or admit to, insecurity of the knee 'My knee gives way' or 'feels as if it will give way'. This is *not* gross insecurity of late-stage OA when the joint ligaments are all loose and there is gross bony deformity. This insecurity is a common complaint in early OA and may greatly limit the patient's activities because of the fear of the joint giving way and being 'made a fool of' when out in company or shopping. It is probably due to muscle weakness, which may be present even in very early disease.

Crepitus

This joint 'noise' can be felt with the hand on the knee. Some patients are very aware of crepitus and it is this symptom that brings these patients to the GP. The more severe the joint damage, the more prolonged the crepitus. It may be a feature of any joint with OA, though it is more difficult to appreciate in hand joints. Crepitus can occasionally be heard as well as felt, and this is more likely in the more severely affected joints.

Can crepitus occur in normal joints? Crepitus can occur in joints that are not being used normally. It also occurs in people who have not used a joint for some time, for instance following the removal of a plaster cast on a leg or arm. The adjacent joints are invariably normal. Crepitus will be present until the joint has become fully mobile again. Crepitus is sometimes associated with sports or minor injuries to tendons or muscles around a joint, as well as injuries to a joint itself. Crepitus tends to be of a minor degree and disappears as the injury heals. It is possible that crepitus only appears in a joint that moves slowly in comparison to a normal joint. These examples suggest that crepitus occurs in joints that have not developed OA but it is a constant symptom/sign of osteo-arthritic joints.

General symptoms in patients with osteoarthritis

As well as looking at and examining the individual joints that the patient complains of, it is important to consider the patient as a whole. General symptoms such as lack of mobility and the inability to perform certain everyday tasks, often lead to frustration and increasing social isolation which can cause mild depression and this will certainly affect the overall management.

Fear or anxiety about the future—even the fear of the imminent need for a wheelchair—have a profound effect on pain. If not addressed in an early consultation, this may lead to failure of management, or even to a patient not returning to the GP and not seeking any further medical advice, or possibly seeking inappropriate advice elsewhere. Importantly, remember OA develops slowly over months and years. An elderly patient may present with early disease and other comorbidities such as diabetes, obesity and hypertension. The development and progression of the arthritis may be the insult that has produced the disability or the social isolation that now requires a holistic approach to the patient's management.

Summary points

- Take a good case history and examine the patient.
- Always exclude 'Red Flags'.
- Pattern recognition aids diagnosis.
- Hip pain may be referred to the knee.
- Emotion affects pain.
- Muscle weakness may be present in early OA.
- Comorbidities must be considered.
- Pseudogout affects people over 70.

References

1 Waddell G, Feder G, McIntosh A, Lewis M, Hutchinson A. *Clinical Guidelines for the Management of Acute Low Back Pain.* London: Royal College of General Practitioners, 1996.
2 Dieppe PA, Doherty M, MacFarlane DG, Maddison PJ. *Rheumatological Medicine.* London: Churchill Livingstone, 1985.

CHAPTER 4

Examination of Joints

A good history is essential in primary care, and in most situations the amount of information that can be gained from an examination over and above that obtained from a good history is limited.

Why examine the joint?

- To exclude 'Red Flags'.
- To exclude referred pain, e.g. from hip disease, as a cause of knee pain.
- Patients may expect to be examined and the reassurance provided by a hands-on examination of the joint followed by a positive feedback (report) to the patient may be better than that provided by an unnecessary X-ray.
- Sometimes we are surprised by what we find! This may be from a negative as well as a positive concept.
- It is becoming more important to record this examination as it provides a ready reckoner for an easy assessment of likely disabilities and handicaps and if, and how, they have changed over time. If we are going to refer our patients for advice from orthopaedic surgeons or to social services, physiotherapy or occupational therapy, we must ensure that we are using scarce resources wisely.

This more detailed examination may take time, which is not available in every consultation. It will depend upon the length of history taking and the joint or joints involved, but examination must be undertaken at some stage, preferably at the initial consultation. With practice and use of a quick refined examination procedure, even restricted to one area, e.g. upper or lower limbs, a great deal may be discovered (see Appendix 1 for 'GALS' technique).

Detailed examination

Look

If possible, observe the patient walking into the consulting room. Osteoarthritic joints tend to be swollen, although usually only slightly.

Some, e.g. the acromioclavicular joints, may look particularly swollen. Swelling of osteoarthritis (OA) joints makes the joints look squarer. The cause may be as follows.

- Mild bony swelling due to the marginal osteophytes giving an altered contour to the joint ('squaring of the joint').
- Mild inflammation.
- Sometimes, especially in the knees, there may be a small effusion.
- Enlarged medial fat pads in knees of elderly patients.

Warning

If there is a large effusion or a hot joint, suggesting a lot of inflammation, be suspicious and exclude a more serious disorder (see 'Red Flags', Chapter 3, pp. 19–21).

In the knee, look for quadriceps wasting. It can be difficult to detect in the elderly patient. This wasting is much more easily seen than measured. If there is no wasting, even in early disease, it is unlikely that there is any significant knee pathology. Comparing both sides helps if only one knee is affected. If both are affected, usually one is worse than the other. This is often the patient's lead leg, i.e. the one that initiates movement. In patients with more severe disease there may be some deformity such as a mild flexion deformity, or a varus angulation (see Fig. 2.8, p. 16).

Usually, patients initially present with complaints about joints on their dominant side, even when the OA is affecting the clavicular joints.

Large joints

Hip disease

In hip disease there may be a fixed flexion deformity of the hip so that the patient limps. This is often seen as an antalgic gait where the patient hurries off the hip joint because of pain. This can be confirmed on examination of the patient. The patient lies on the couch and flexes the good hip (normal flexion is 135°). If there is loss of flexion in the other hip, then this thigh lifts from the couch and the knee will also flex. This is called a Thomas test (Fig. 4.1).

Pain-causing weakness of the hip abductors so that the pelvis on the unaffected (opposite) side drops when the patient's weight is on the diseased hip. This is called a Trendelenburg gait. The Trendelenburg test for weak abductors is illustrated in Fig. 4.2.

Naturally, there may be a mixture of these gaits. A rolling gait or nautical roll is a mixed Trendelenburg and antalgic gait. Here, both hips

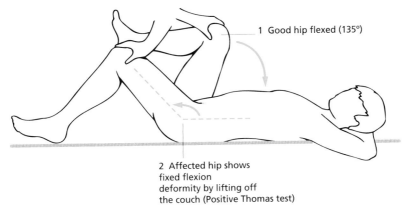

1 Good hip flexed (135°)

2 Affected hip shows
fixed flexion
deformity by lifting off
the couch (Positive Thomas test)

Fig. 4.1 Thomas test. Perform manoeuvre 1. If action 2 is observed the test is positive. From [1] with permission.

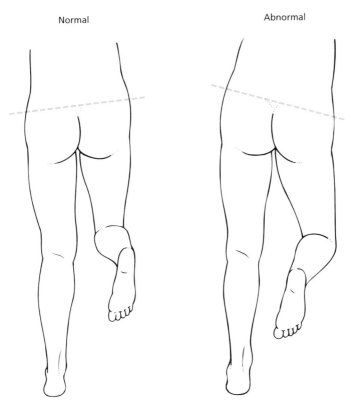

Normal

Abnormal

Fig. 4.2 Trendelenburg test for weak abductors. Patient stands on one leg. If opposite hip abductors are weak then the pelvis tilts away from the standing leg. From [1] with permission.

are affected so both have shortened stand phases and a pelvic tilt on both sides from weak abductors. In a waddling gait there is severe weakness of the abductors. Hip replacements that are becoming loose, or ones which have been aligned too horizontally, may cause this.

Knee disease

A few patients will present with obvious bow legs. They usually have severe OA and, on closer inspection, there may be squaring of the joint and an effusion. This is varus deformity (see Fig. 2.8). Valgus deformity is commoner in patients with inflammatory arthritis, e.g. rheumatoid arthritis or pseudogout.

Feel

The joints affected may seem harder or larger than the normal comparator and the joint may feel as if it is closer to the skin's surface. It may be tender along the joint line or there may be tender areas around the joint. These tender points are usually present in early OA and palpation of the joint should include palpation for these.

Patients with knee OA almost universally have pain on palpation over the area of the anserine bursa, as shown in Figs 4.3 and 4.4.

This tender point has been known about for centuries and is the spleen 9 line shown in Chinese acupuncture charts. A clinical effusion may be present in severe OA but this is unlikely in patients with mild to moderate OA.

In most large joints with OA it is possible to 'feel' crepitus (see Chapter 3). Demonstrating that we as primary care doctors can feel this crepitus is part of patient education and it helps to develop empathy with the patient. We may already be quite certain of the diagnosis from the patient's history. We are undertaking a more detailed examination when we elicit crepitus and check for joint movements and even speed of movements. We will be trying to identify if the patient's pain comes from within the joint, around the joint or from the joint line.

Move

There is no hard-and-fast rule when moving joints that the movements should be active or passive. Different examiners have different priorities and evolve a system with which they are comfortable—the essential priority is to examine each patient appropriately.

Moving affected joints through their range of movements may give

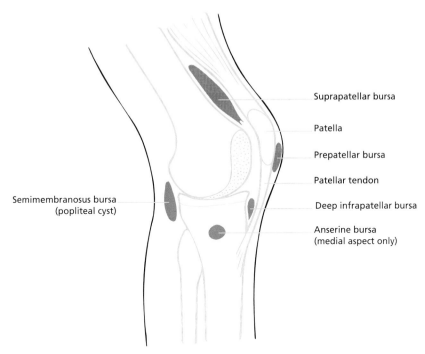

Suprapatellar bursa

Patella

Prepatellar bursa

Patellar tendon

Deep infrapatellar bursa

Anserine bursa
(medial aspect only)

Semimembranosus bursa
(popliteal cyst)

Fig. 4.3

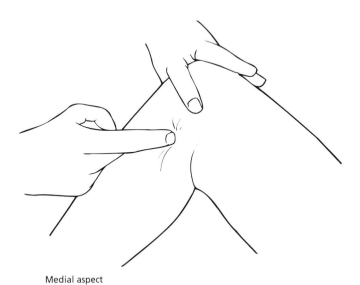

Medial aspect

Fig. 4.4 Common periarticular tender site: (L) index over joint line (R) index over insertion of medial collateral ligament.

4

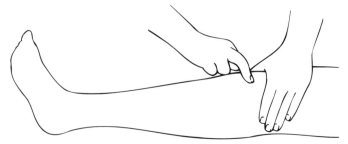

Fig. 4.5 Patella tap test (for moderate or large effusions). From [1] with permission.

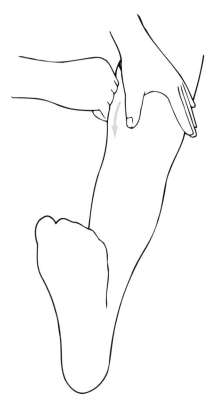

Fig. 4.6 Cross fluctuation test (for small effusions). From [1] with permission.

- Patella tap test (for moderate to larger effusions). With your non-dominant hand, squash the fluid from the suprapatella pouch to behind the patella (Fig. 4.5). Use a finger or thumb of your dominant hand to ballotte the patella on to the femur below. This will give an indication of the amount of fluid in the joint.
- Cross fluctuation test (swipe or bulge test). Stabilize the patella with one hand (using your thumb) (Fig. 4.6). Empty the medial compartment of the knee joint by stroking downwards on the medial aspect. The fluid

should flow to the lateral gutter. In one movement, with the patella still stabilized by your thumb, stroke or push on the lateral side and look for a bulge on the medial aspect. This test is more sensitive for smaller effusions than the patella tap test (Fig. 4.5).

What may confuse the clinical picture?

In patients who have inflammation (synovitis) of the joint capsule and synovial linings the 'bogginess' can be mistaken for a small to moderate effusion. This is more likely in patients with active synovitis from rheumatoid arthritis than in patients with OA. Elderly women often have large medial fat pads, which may be mistaken for effusions. These fat pads are tender on palpation; chronic effusions are not.

Occasionally, a patient may present with a large, tense but cool effusion that is difficult to examine because of knee pain. It is sensible to ask for advice urgently from secondary care.

Further examinations and assessments

The next assessment is the range of movement and speed of movement (as well as feeling for any crepitus). This can be undertaken with the patient sitting on the edge of a couch or sometimes on a chair. Passive movement (the examiner moving the relaxed joint) may feel slightly stiff and slower when compared to the normal knee or the less affected knee. Check for fixed flexion by assessing any gap between the back of the knee and the couch when the patient is lying on his or her back. At the same time, any popliteal cysts may be felt. Often this is an incidental finding but it may be worrying the patient. In younger patients especially (but not exclusively) check for knee hypermobility (genu recurvatum). This is best done with the patient standing; if present, remember to look for other signs of hypermobility (see Appendix 3 for Beighton's score). Hypermobility tends to precipitate many musculoskeletal consultations and problems, as there are more ligamentous sprains and strains and probably a higher incidence of OA in previous hypermobile joints.

Knee joint stability

Patients may present for the first time in primary care with gross OA with knee joints that are very unstable. Sometimes they have a flare of their underlying OA due to some mild trauma, such as a stumble walking across cobblestones or an awkward turn. The presentation may be

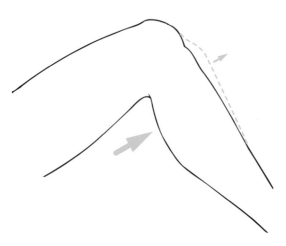

Fig. 4.7 Anterior draw test to test for anterior cruciate integrity. From [1] with permission.

because of giving way, or the feeling of giving way. There may be a small of large effusion—how do we assess these patients?
• Check extension, flexion and speed of movement and compare both sides.
• Check forward–backward stability, i.e. the draw test (see below), checking for excessive movement at the tibiofemoral joint. These movements are controlled by the anterior and posterior cruciate ligaments (ACL and PCL).

The draw test (Fig. 4.7)

The patient lies supine on a couch with the hip flexed at 45° and knee at 90°. The examiner places his or her hands posteriorly behind the tibia and exerts a forward pull. Too much movement means instability and probably a ruptured ACL (anterior draw test).

Push the tibia posteriorly—if there is too much movement here this suggests a ruptured PCL (positive posterior draw test).

Explained like this, the draw test seems an easy test to perform and interpret. This may be so in grossly unstable knees but in younger patients and in athletes with strong muscles, all tests for cruciate ligament and meniscal problems are fraught with difficulties and even experienced orthopaedic surgeons, using a battery of examination tests, do not invariably make the correct diagnosis. It would appear that few primary care doctors see enough patients to become experts in these tests and maintain this proficiency. It is suggested that a good history, examination for pain, a draw test and checking the integrity of the collateral ligaments will usually allow primary care doctors to judge when further investigations or opinions are necessary.

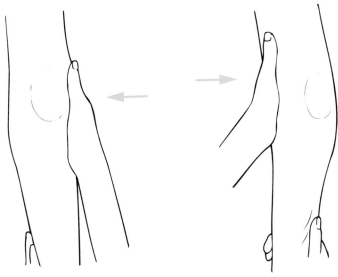

Fig. 4.8 Testing collateral ligament intergrity. Lateral pressure is applied to a slightly flexed knee to see if it will rock from side to side.

Test for collateral ligament integrity

When assessing a patient's medial and lateral collateral ligaments, the knee should be flexed to about 30° so that the posterior capsule and PCL are relaxed.
- The patient lies supine on the couch with the heel on the couch and the knee flexed to 30°.
- Lateral stability—apply a force through your palm from the medial aspect of the knee.
- Medial stability—apply a force through your palm from the lateral aspect of the knee.
- Remember to compare with the other side.

This assessment is illustrated in Fig. 4.8.

In patients with gross OA, any instability is very often painless, or relatively so (this is not so in an athlete), but it is still usually the cause of the knee giving way or the feeling of giving way. Remember, in early OA, that a feeling of giving way is probably due to muscle weakness.

Meniscal problems

Meniscal injuries may occur to anyone performing an activity that involves rotation and/or physical contact. The greatest number occur in young athletes but may occur at any age and in joints which already

Table 4.1 Examination check list for knee diagnosis.

Knee problem	Symptoms			
	Pain	Swelling	Giving way	Locking
Osteoarthritis	✓	✓	✓ (advanced)	✓ (if loose bodies)
Rheumatoid arthritis	✓	✓	✓ (advanced)	
Gout/pseudogout	✓	✓		
Direct trauma	✓	✓	✓	
Meniscal problems	✓	✓	✓	✓
Loose body	✓	✓	✓	✓
Anterior knee pain	✓	✓	Possibly	
Bursitis	✓	✓		Rarely (if cartilage debris)

show signs of osteoarthritis. (For meniscal injuries and development of osteoarthritis, see Chapter 9.)

What may make you suspect meniscal problems?
- Locking.
- Limited extension.
- An effusion—acute or recurrent.
- Grating rather than crepitus.
- Quadriceps wasting—especially in young athletes.
- Joint line tenderness—which may be present at different degrees of flexion (see Chapter 3).

If the patient has any of the problems listed above, then referral is required for further investigations, such as MRI or arthroscopy, to assess the internal joint damage. There are no hard-and-fast rules as to which of these investigations is correct. The way forward is often on a practical basis, that is consideration of the individual patient, local expertise, primary care access to MRI and the length of the arthroscopy waiting list. Further availability of real time MRI video recordings may play a part in the future.

Table 4.1 summarizes the differential diagnosis for knee pain from clinical signs and symptoms.

The hip

In osteoarthritis of the hip, the pain, classically, is felt anteriorly in the groin around the femoral triangle, lateral to the femoral artery, but may be periarticular over the lateral thigh, buttock or referred to the front of the thigh and knee. See Fig. 4.9 which illustrates these areas of pain.

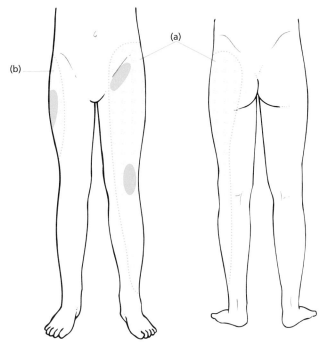

Fig. 4.9 Areas where pain may radiate for (a) hip OA and (b) trochanteric bursitis. Dark shading denotes classical areas of pain; light shading less common or less intense areas of pain. From [2] with permission.

Trochanteric bursitis (Figs 4.9 and 4.10)

Periarticular structures causing pain in hip disease are invariably the trochanteric bursae. The pain involves the superficial trochanteric bursa in the majority of patients and is shown in Fig. 4.10.

The maximum point of pain is often subtrochanteric on the lateral aspect of the thigh and if the patient is standing, this is at the level of the pubic symphysis. It is assumed that the cause is related to the extra stress put on the hip external rotators when internal rotation of the hip is limited. It is this movement (internal rotation) that is the first to be lost in hip OA and occurs before loss of hip flexion.

Deep trochanteric bursitis (see Fig. 4.10) may also occur especially if the patient has fallen. Very often the fall is related to osteoarthritis present in the hip or knee. The pain may cause a limp (antalgic gait). The pain is usually deep and burning, or just a severe ache and worse at night, especially when lying on the affected side.

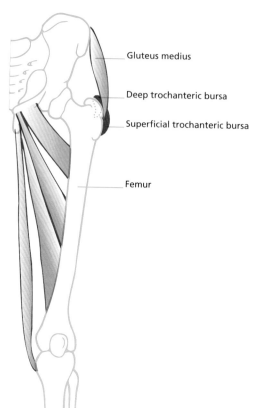

Fig. 4.10 Trochanteric bursae, superficial and deep. From [1] with permission.

Gluteus medius

Deep trochanteric bursa

Superficial trochanteric bursa

Femur

Examination of the hip

The best way to examine hips is by using an examination couch with the patient lying supine, preferably with trousers or tights removed. The movements essential to undertake are internal rotation and flexion.

Internal rotation, as already stated, is the first movement to be restricted in OA of the hip. Flex the hip to 90° and bend the knee to a right angle, then using the foot as a pointer, rotate the leg away from the body, so moving/rotating the head of the femur internally. Normal internal rotation is 35° and external rotation 45°. This is shown in Fig. 4.11.

We must also check flexion, which is normally 135° and may be assessed by bending the knee and pushing the thigh up to the patient's chest.

It is possible to check passive hip rotation with the patient sitting on the edge of the couch. The patient sits on the couch so that the knees are at right angles and feet above the floor (see Fig. 4.12). The patient puts the hands on the hips so that the examiner will be able to notice at what

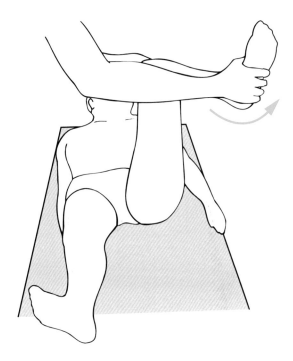

Fig. 4.11 Internal rotation of the hip. (Patient supine method.)

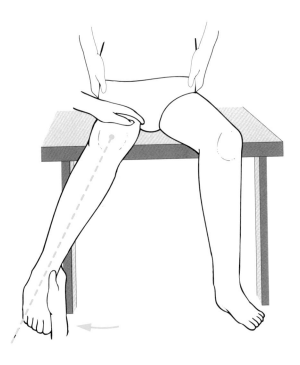

Fig. 4.12 Assessing internal rotation of the hip: patient sitting method. The patient should sit with legs free from the floor (e.g. over the end of a couch). Stabilize the thigh with one hand. Grip lower end of tibia and rotate the whole limb externally (to show internal rotation of the hip joint) and internally (to show external rotation of the hip joint). From the PCR Hip Study.

point the hip begins to rise (this is the limit of internal rotation). The examiner places one hand on the patient's thigh to steady it and holds the patient's ankle with the other hand. This hand then moves the patient's leg away from the central line. The distance the foot moves from this central line gives the arc of the rotation, so that the angle traversed may be judged (normally 35°). A less sensitive assessment may be made with the patient sitting on a chair. Unfortunately, most chairs are just too low for an accurate assessment to be made. Remember that even this is better than no assessment and may be extended to a further examination immediately, or at a later consultation. This examination may help in reducing overall reliance on the X-ray for clinical decisions. Normal internal rotation is almost incompatible with OA hip.

We have already considered the Thomas test for a fixed flexion deformity. Occasionally, patients present so late that they have bilateral fixed flexion deformity of the hips. They will be unable to lie flat on the examination couch and may present with sleeping problems if they have not had hip pain severe enough to consult in the first place. In primary care it is amazing what may present for the first time.

The clavicular joints

Osteoarthritis of the acromioclavicular joint

Patients usually complain of pain on shoulder movement. Initially, in primary care, we may not suspect acromioclavicular (AC) joint arthritis as part of a mixed picture of a painful arc or shoulder capsulitis (see Fig. 4.13).

Be suspicious of AC joint OA if the patient cannot raise the arm laterally to perform a full arc. In the classical scenario the patient is unable to raise the arm above the pain. Unfortunately, in many patients there is not a clear-cut picture. Very often the AC joint pain has limited all shoulder movement resulting in the patient's inability to perform a full arc examination, or to fully externally rotate their glenohumeral joint and put a hand behind their head, because of limited abduction and elevation (see Fig. 4.13).

Patients usually point to the AC joint
Palpation over the joint produces local tenderness
Painful at extreme of arc, i.e. unable to 'get' above the pain (cf. subacromial bursitis)
Painful if arm moved across chest towards other shoulder

Table 4.2 Signs that produce pain in AC joint disease.

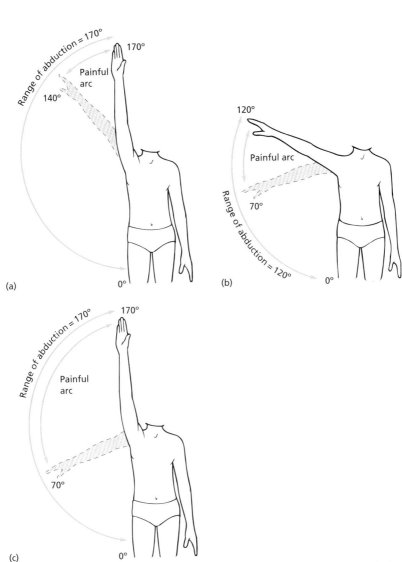

Fig. 4.13 (a) Painful arc: acromioclavicular joint—painful arc; pain is experienced in the last 30° of abduction or flexion, so unable to 'get above the pain'. Pain is also produced when the arms are moved across the chest (so-called scarf test). (b) Capsulitis—painful arc; pain is experienced in the terminal range of abduction with restricted shoulder movements especially elevation restriction (subacromial painful arc—mid arc pain and able to 'get above the pain'). (c) Composite painful arc; this is common in the older population. Pain experienced over a large arc of abduction and not able to 'get above the pain' or too painful to attempt. There are many variations of this depending upon the different pathologies involved and the overall quality of the shoulder muscles. From [3] by permission of Oxford University Press.

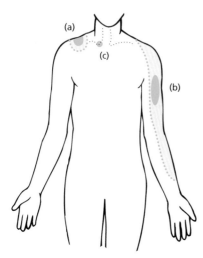

Fig. 4.14 Patterns of pain around the shoulder area involved for (a) the acromioclavicular joint, (b) the glenohumeral joint and (c) the sternoclavicular joint. From [2] by permission of Oxford University Press.

Remember to palpate over the AC joint. In OA of the AC joint palpation over the joint may elicit considerable tenderness and reproduce the patient's pain. This pain may also be referred down the arm as well as around the joint (see Fig. 4.14). Always ask your patient to extend the arm across the chest towards the other shoulder—this will be very painful and invariably present in AC joint pathology (scarf test).

Sternoclavicular joint

OA of this joint occurs quite commonly. Very few of these patients are referred on for a secondary care opinion. The patient may present because they have noticed a swollen tender area, which may also be warm to the touch. This scenario of warmth, swelling and pain is extremely worrying to patients who may seriously consider that they have a tumour and they require the good counselling of their primary care doctor. The pain is not referred anywhere, nor do there appear to be any periarticular points of pain.

The differential diagnosis will be a subluxation caused by trauma, such as a motor vehicle accident or a sprain from unusual activity. Rarer conditions are involvement in rheumatoid arthritis, a tumour, or metabolic diseases (such as a hyperostosis). Remember 'Red Flags'—any joint may become infected.

Metatarsophalangeal joint

X-ray evidence of arthritis at the metatarsophalangeal joint is very common but this joint is often painless unless exposed to an insult when the

Table 4.3 Qualities of footwear for all patients with OA.

- Thick soft sole (shock absorbing)
- No raised heel
- Broad forefoot (especially if a hallux valgus is present)
- Deep soft uppers
- Arch support (preferably of sorbothane)
- Shoes with secure fastenings. No slip-ons.

4

pain produced seems to lead to a flare of the arthritis affecting the joint. The insult can be something as simple as stubbing a toe. The joint may become warmer and give pain on activity that may last for a few days longer than the patient might expect. Quite often it is this prolonged period of pain that brings the patient to the primary care doctor. There will be pain on palpation, and pain on passive movement of the joint, so that there may well be a hallux rigidus from the muscle spasm. This gradually resolves. The differential diagnosis is from acute gout, which needs to be excluded (see Chapter 3).

In severely affected joints, it may be the additional features that bring the patient (e.g. an overlying bunion on the hallux valgus, Fig. 4.15) problems with the over-riding toes or a fixed hallux rigidus, so that the patient finds the big toe painful and stiff on walking. Nearly all patients presenting to their primary care doctor in this situation will be wearing inappropriate shoes. It is extremely rare to see people with these problems who are already wearing shock-absorbing, wide fitting shoes such as trainers, or the equivalent proprietary shoes.

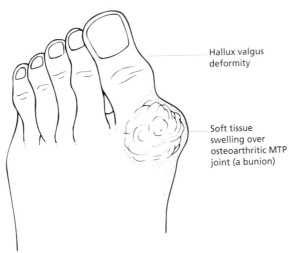

Hallux valgus
deformity

Soft tissue
swelling over
osteoarthritic MTP
joint (a bunion)

Fig. 4.15 Hallux valgus deformity. A soft tissue swelling (a bunion) over an osteoarthritic metatarsophalangeal joint. From [4] with permission.

4

The spine

Osteoarthritis, by definition, only affects synovial joints. Synovial joints in the spine are called the apophyseal or facet joints. The cervical and lumbar intervertebral joints undergo degenerative changes with disc space narrowing, osteophytes, and even disc protrusions. It is unclear what the relationship is between the intervertebral and facet joints. Patients having such changes in their spine may have varying symptoms and pain, from nothing or a slight twinge to quite severe pain. The pain may be aggravated by movement and standing. X-rays on these patients often show degenerative changes, but despite such findings, most patients have mechanical back pain and would be best managed as suggested in the *RCGP Back Pain Guidelines* [5]. Very often there is referred or radiating pain as well as local areas of pain close to the spine.

Back pain examination does not help differentiate between articular pain and periarticular pain. In considering back pain, as with joint pain, it is essential to exclude 'Red Flags' and perform a diagnostic triage (as described in the *RCGP Back Pain Guidelines*).

If diagnostic triage is undertaken and 'Red Flags' are excluded, then the overall diagnostic label of mechanical backache is appropriate and treatment may be directed towards mobilization and increasing activity. Just as in other forms of OA, we need to encourage exercise, both general and specific. This is much more helpful for patients than labelling them with degenerative disease or OA as these terms tend to imply and engender a negative and regressive approach to management, both by the primary care doctor and in terms of self-management by the patient.

The American College of Rheumatology (ACR) [6,7,8] has produced guidelines for the diagnosis of osteoarthritis at various sites. These guidelines were produced for clinical research and population based studies. The guidelines help identify patients who are at the more severe end of the spectrum. The essential criteria is joint pain for most days of the month and to this has to be added clinical bony enlargement (squaring) of the joint or X-ray changes of OA. See Table 4.4; these are modified criteria for the knee.

Use of these criteria would include the 10% of patients who will have been referred, or require secondary care, perhaps including surgery. It certainly leaves out the vast majority of patients. The criteria define the diagnosis, but they do not help assess how our patients are coping with their osteoarthritis. We will consider this assessment in Chapter 5.

Table 4.4 ACR guidelines for diagnosing clinical OA of the knee [9].

1	Knee pain for most days of the month
2	Crepitus on active joint motion
3	Morning stiffness of less than 30 min in duration
4	Age over 38 years
5	Bony enlargement of the knee on examination

OA present if 1, 2, 3, 4 present
Or 1 and 5 present

Primary care diagnosis of OA—summary

- Pattern recognition gives a presumptive diagnosis.
- History and discussion increases confidence in the presumptive diagnosis.
- Examination for shape, pain, crepitus and movement usually confirms the diagnosis.
- Blood tests and X-rays are rarely helpful.

Summary points

- Exclude 'Red Flags' by examination.
- Crepitus can be felt.
- Quadriceps wasting can be seen or felt.
- OA causes bow legs (varus).
- Think of pseudogout if patient has valgus and a painful knee.
- OA causes slowing of joint movement.
- Anterior knee pain is worse when descending stairs.
- Trochanteric bursitis can be an added cause of hip pain.
- Shock absorbing shoes are helpful for OA.

References

1 *Diploma in Primary Care Rheumatology, Module 5 lower limb*, University of Bath, Department of Continuing and Distance Education.
2 Brandt KD, Doherty M, Lohmander LS. *Osteoarthritis*. Oxford: Oxford University Press, 1998.
3 Hutson MA. *Sports Injuries: Recognition and Management*. Oxford: Oxford University Press, 1990.
4 Dieppe PA, Doherty M, MacFarlane DG, Maddison PJ. *Rheumatological Medicine*. London: Churchill Livingstone, 1985.

5   Waddell G, Feder G, McIntosh A, Lewis M, Hutchinson A. *Clinical Guidelines for the Management of Acute Low Back Pain*. Royal College of General Practitioners Report, 1996.

6   Altman R, Alarcon G, Appelrouth D *et al*. The American College of Rheumatology (ACR) Criteria for the Classification and Reporting of Osteoarthritis of the hip. *Arthritis & Rheumatism* 1991; 34 (5): 505–14.

7   Altman R, Alarcon G, Appelrouth D *et al*. The American College of Rheumatology criteria for the classification of osteoarthritis of the hand. *Arthritis Rheum* 1990; 33 (11): 1601–10.

8   Altman R, Asch E, Bloch D *et al*. The American College of Rheumatology criteria for the classification of osteoarthritis of the knee. Diagnostic and Therapeuric Criteria Committee of the American Rheumatism Association. *Arthritis Rheum* 1986; 29 (8): 1039–49.

9   Silman AJ, Hochberg MC. *Epidemiology of the Rheumatic Diseases*. Oxford: Oxford University Press, 1993.

4

CHAPTER 5

Assessment of Osteoarthritis Including Hand Osteoarthritis

Everyone copes with problems in different ways and all to a varying ability. Treatment of any medical condition should be 'patient centred' and not 'disease focused'. This being said, how should osteoarthritis (OA) be assessed?

There are three elements of assessment (Fig. 5.1), all relating to the patient.

- Pain—how does this affect the patient?
- Function—what has happened to work, home and leisure?
- Joint damage—what is happening to the joint?

Why is this classification important?

Assessment and classification of OA into mild, moderate and severe has allowed the development of a range of treatments and management strategies. These include education, prevention, medical interventions, surgical management and aftercare. Importantly, we are able to consider educational programmes for the population that may have OA but never seek, or stop seeking, help and advice.

Pain

As in Chapter 3, this chapter discusses pain and how it is an essential element of the clinical diagnosis of OA.

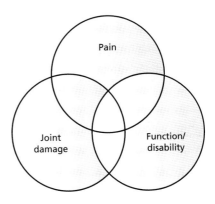

Fig. 5.1 Each of the elements may have an impact on the patient to varying degrees and all may or may not overlap and interrelate. For example, a patient's X-ray may show structural change but this may not be reflected in his or her pain and function.

Definition of pain (based on the international definition)

Pain is an unpleasant sensory and emotional experience associated with actual, or potential, tissue damage, or described in terms of such damage. Pain is always subjective. Each individual learns the application of the word through experience related to injury in early life. It is always unpleasant and therefore also an emotional experience.

We know what *we* mean by mild pain but perception of it by our patients and colleagues may differ. Categories of mild, moderate and severe pain need some clarification. Importantly, the international definition of pain includes emotion as a major component and allows empathy with our patients.

Mild pain

Little or no pain in the joints, but some discomfort and episodes of pain may occur at irregular intervals, usually related to activities; sometimes only one specific activity.

Moderate pain

Severity of pain becomes intrusive and/or disruptive in a significant proportion of daily activities.

Severe pain

Pain has a major adverse effect on simple, essential daily activities, such as walking short distances, as well as on work, sleep and hobbies.

The American College of Rheumatology (ACR) has included only one level of pain in the ACR definition of OA—pain for most days of the prior month (see Chapter 4, Table 4.4 [5,6,7]). This defines patients who definitely do have OA and is appropriate when patients are being included, or enrolled, into clinical trials and research. It does not include a lot of patients seen in primary care with milder degrees of OA and may not be helpful in applying strategies for limiting progression or applying secondary preventions.

Function

We need to assess how OA is affecting the patient's everyday life. This ranges from hardly affecting to totally affecting the patient's quality of life. A simple (mild/moderate/severe) classification will allow us to record this assessment so we will be able to assess over time as long as we remember to record every patient contact and our findings. We should try to record a simple function classification at each patient encounter.

Mild functional impairment

Patients are able to undertake most, if not all, essential everyday tasks as well as hobbies and leisure activities with little difficulty or significant need for help.

Moderate functional impairment

Some recreational, leisure or work activities are significantly disrupted by the joint problems resulting in some need for help (or aids) without which activities are impossible.

Severe functional impairment

Joint function has a major effect on social and recreational activities as well as on everyday life and tasks. Patients in this category require a lot of help and usually require aids. Many things about life are impossible.

Joint damage

Pain and function have been assessed clinically. In the majority of patients, joint damage should be assessed clinically. Clinical evaluation of damage ranges from crepitus only and minimal restrictions of movement, through to squaring of the joint and gross restriction of movements, with or without effusions, to major deformities and instability. There is no specific need for an X-ray. Although most patients with significant OA will have had the joint X-rayed at some stage, over-reliance on X-rays for clinical decisions should be avoided. X-ray changes will range from a normal joint through to osteophytes, bone cysts and sclerosis, to total loss of joint space.

Mild joint damage

Crepitus will usually, but not invariably, be felt on joint movement. Squaring of the joint may be apparent or it may just feel harder and slightly larger than a normal joint. As the disease progresses, passive movement of the joint may be slightly slower than normal. X-rays of the joint may be reported as normal or may show osteophytes and little else. Joint space narrowing is either absent or very mild. X-rays of knee joints must be taken in the weight-bearing position.

Moderate joint damage

In these patients both active and passive movements are slow, restricted and painful with crepitus and joint squaring. There may also be an effusion. Weight-bearing X-rays of knees will show definite joint space narrowing, as well as osteophytes, and there may be sclerosis and changes in subchondral bone.

Severe joint damage

These patients will have clinical evidence of obvious deformity, often varus or fixed flexion deformity. There may be joint instability. Weight-bearing X-rays of knees should show complete or almost total loss of cartilage (shown on X-rays as joint space narrowing) in at least one compartment, with or without bone damage, plus features seen in moderate joint damage.

Validated formal assessments

We have been discussing a simple clinical assessment that is quick and practical. Sometimes a more structured assessment is required, this may be for clinical reasons or because of an audit or research requirements. Two well-validated instruments are available for OA. The Lequesne index for hip and knee OA is usually administered by a doctor or an observer. The Western Ontario and MacMaster Universities Osteoarthritis Index (WOMAC) was developed and validated by Professor Nicolas Bellamy. It is a self-administered questionnaire (i.e. by the patient, see Appendix 1). The original questionnaire copyright was for knees and hips; recently, he has developed one for hand OA [1,2].

Table 5.1 shows this classification diagrammatically and how it is really a continuum, though an individual patient may not progress or may even improve. Naturally, patients may present for the first time at any point in the disease process.

Table 5.1 Assessment of OA relates diagnosis to effect on the patient.

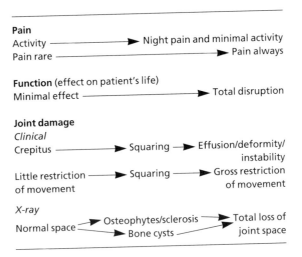

5

Summary points

- Making a diagnosis in OA is only the beginning. We must assess how the individual is being affected.
- Assessing pain, function and joint damage helps to decide management strategies.
- Over-reliance on X-rays for clinical decision making should be avoided.
- The WOMAC and Lequesne questionnaires may be used for more formal assessment.

Assessment of hand osteoarthritis

Patients visit their doctor when they have noticed problems with their hands. A common presentation is with acute, hot Heberden's nodes (or Bouchard's nodes). As mentioned in Chapter 2, these nodes are a marker for OA *but not of severity*, neither for hand joints nor for the knees. It is very pleasing to be able to say to patients that they are most unlikely to develop joint disease that will be a major problem.

The different patterns of involvement of hand joints (Fig. 5.2) in OA require their own management. In the following classification there are five distinct patterns. There is some debate about whether or not hands go through all the stages from I to V, but there are many patients in primary care who fit well into this type of assessment, who do not change categories and who remain in-type. Most importantly, this assessment

5

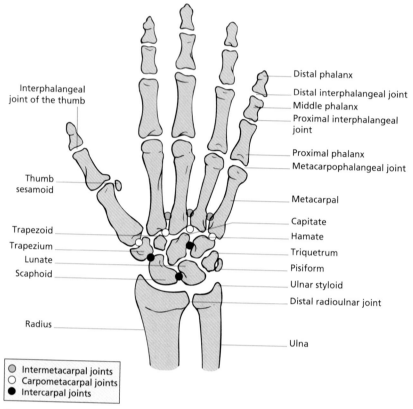

Interphalangeal joint of the thumb

Distal phalanx
Distal interphalangeal joint
Middle phalanx
Proximal interphalangeal joint
Proximal phalanx
Metacarpophalangeal joint

Thumb sesamoid

Metacarpal

Capitate
Hamate
Triquetrum
Pisiform
Ulnar styloid
Distal radioulnar joint

Trapezoid
Trapezium
Lunate
Scaphoid

Radius

Ulna

○ Intermetacarpal joints
○ Carpometacarpal joints
● Intercarpal joints

Fig. 5.2 Bones and joints of the hand and wrist.

by examination, will help primary care doctors in diagnosis and patient management, so leading to improved function and pain control which are major goals of therapy.

Heberden's and Bouchard's nodes

These nodes were described by Heberden as 'little hard knots about the size of a small pea'. They appear on the dorsal aspect of the distal interphalangeal (DIP) joints. Bouchard's nodes are similar but are seen less commonly. They occur on the proximal interphalangeal (PIP) joints. These bony enlargements helped Heberden and Bouchard distinguish OA from other forms of arthritis, e.g. an inflammatory arthritis such as rheumatoid arthritis (RA) and gout. There is a familial occurrence of these nodes with a *strong* female preponderance. There is a debate as to whether the inheritance factor is a single gene or polygenic. Today's evidence suggests the latter.

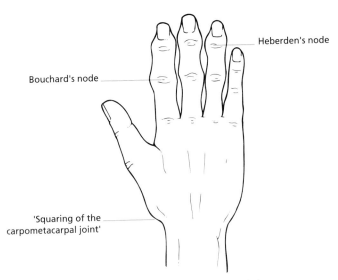

Heberden's node

Bouchard's node

'Squaring of the carpometacarpal joint'

5

Fig. 5.3 Heberden's and Bouchard's nodes. From [3] with permission.

Type I: Heberden's and Bouchard's nodes (Fig. 5.3)

- Patients present with painful Heberden's and/or Bouchard's nodes.
- Nodes painful at times of development only.
- Nodes may be inflamed and very swollen.
- Finger and thumb flexion/extension not affected.
- Minimal loss of function.
- Grip not affected.
- Sometimes in the very elderly, gout may be superimposed on these distal interphalangeal joints—especially if the drug regime includes a thiazide (see Chapter 3).
- Usually, no treatment is required except reassurance. If the nodes are painful and swollen a topical non-steroidal anti-inflammatory drug (NSAID) may be tried. An offer to inject a small volume of steroid into the area of inflammation is rarely accepted.

Type II: squaring of first carpometacarpal thumb joint (Fig. 5.3)

- Patients present with use-related thumb pain.
- There is squaring of the first carpometacarpal (CMC) joint.
- Dominant hand first.
- Grip and grip strength affected.
- Functions for certain actions (twisting grip) painful.
- Other hand joints need not be involved.

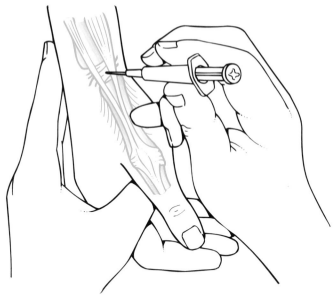

Fig. 5.4 Injections of the thumb base (1st CMC joint). From [4] with permission.

- Responds very well to injection into first CMC joint (Fig. 5.4).
- Resting (thumb) splint useful for night-time pain.

Type III: thick, stiff fingers

- Fingers look wide and thicker, otherwise surprisingly normal.
- May be squaring of DIP, interphalangeal (IP) and metacarpophalangeal (MCP) joints.
- Usually first CMC joints not involved.
- Movements/functions affected by increased tissue in and around flexor sheaths.
- Both hands affected to a varying degree.
- Tight grip on tools or golf clubs difficult; may drop cups.
- Hands very different from those with Dupuytren's contractures.
- May respond to injections into flexor sheaths if seen early enough.

Type IV(a): painful, swollen knuckles

- Patients present with painful MCP joints, especially of index and middle fingers.
- Moderate inflammatory swelling of second and third MCP joints.
- Painful on palpation as well as movement.
- Thumb CMC joints painful and show squaring but are rarely inflamed.

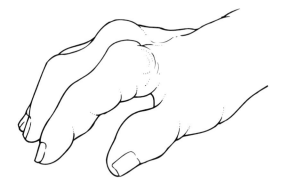

Fig. 5.5 Painful knuckles and thumb. From drawings by Dorothy Tilburn.

- Grip may be severely affected.
- Difficulty with cups, cutlery and buttons (chores).
- Commonly seen in housewives, especially knitters.
- These joints respond well to steroid injections. These injections can be repeated intermittently.

Type IV(b): painful knuckles and thumbs (Fig. 5.5)

- A more florid presentation of type IV(a) described above.
- Most MCP joints and first CMC joints swollen.
- Interphalangeal joints painful and swollen.
- Both hands equally affected.
- Gripping difficult and extremely painful.
- No constitutional upset (in contrast to RA).
- No sweaty palms (in contrast to RA).
- Especially seen in women who work manually (e.g. farmers' wives), but it may affect men.
- Too many joints to inject.
- Most patients respond well to small doses of Salazopyrin (1 g daily) or hydroxychloroquine (200 mg 5 days a week).

Type V: deformed hands—good function (Fig. 5.6)

- These hands show deformities, ulnar deviation of joints and ulnar drift.
- All joints affected.
- Exhibit Heberden's and Bouchard's nodes.
- MCP joints swollen and first CMC joints square.
- Wrist joints may be involved—being painful, or limited movement, or even some ankylosing of joint.
- May be mistaken for RA but:
  1 no severe loss of function as in RA;

5

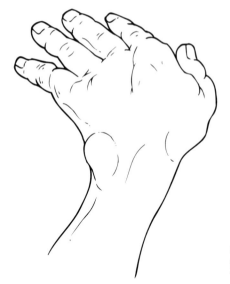

Fig. 5.6 Deformed hands: good function. From drawings by Dorothy Tilburn.

2 retain strong hand and thumb grip;
3 flares of joints caused by knocks from manual work;
4 analgesics or an appropriately placed injection are required for flares;
5 inflammatory markers are negative.

What may confuse the clinical picture?

- Sometimes the joints of type V hands become unstable.
- X-ray report—this may state that there are erosions in unstable DIP joints. OA erosions are central in OA, not peripheral as in RA, but the report may not categorize them. If possible, view the X-rays, or ask for clarification, to avoid erroneous diagnosis and treatment.

Summary points

- Heberden's nodes are not a marker of severity.
- Major loss of hand function is rare in OA.
- Injections into thumb base often produce long periods of pain relief.
- Beware of incorrectly interpreting reported erosions in OA hands.
- Hands can suffer from inflammatory OA.

References

1 Lequesne MG, Mery C, Samson M *et al.* Indexes of severity for osteoarthritis of the hip and knee: validation—Value in comparison with other assessment tests. *Scand J Rheumatol* 1987 (Suppl. 65): 85–9.

2 Bellamy N, Buchanan WW, Goldsmith CH *et al.* Validation Study of WOMAC: A health status instrument for measuring clinically important patient relevant outcomes to antirheumatic drug therapy in patients with osteoarthritis of the hip or knee. *J Rheumatol* 1988 15: 1833–40.

3 Dieppe PA, Doherty M, MacFarlane DG, Maddison PJ. *Rheumatological Medicine*. Edinburgh: Churchill Livingstone, 1985.

4 Silver, T. *Joint and Soft Tissue Injections*. Abingdon: Radcliffe Medical Press, 1998.

5 Altman R, Alarcon G, Appelrouth D *et al.* The American College of Rheumatology for the classification and reporting of osteoarthritis of the hip. *Arthritis Rheum* 1991; 34 (5): 505–14.

6 Altman R, Alarcon G, Appelrouth D *et al.* The American College of Rheumatology criteria for the classification of osteoarthritis of the hand. *Arthritis Rheum* 1990; 33 (11): 1601–10.

7 Altman R, Asch E, Bloch D *et al.* The American College of Rheumatology criteria for the classification of osteoarthritis of the knee. Diagnostic and Therapeutic Criteria Committee of the American Rheumatism Association. *Arthritis Rheum* 1986; 29 (8): 1039–49.

5

Management Options—Education, Behavioural and Environmental

Education

Education is vital in the management of a condition such as osteoarthritis (OA), not only for doctors but also for patients and the general public. The more the public and patients know about OA and understand the condition, the more they will be able to help themselves and know when to seek professional help.

Patient education

Pain is the usual presenting symptom for patients with OA and they come to their doctors for help in dealing with this. Explanation, education, counselling and lifestyle advice will be all that is required for some patients, together with a full explanation of the use of a simple analgesic such as paracetamol (acetaminophen). Patient expectations, however, often include the idea that they must have a drug treatment, almost to validate their problem, and it may take considerable persuasion by the doctor, over many consultations, to encourage the patient to try non-drug measures.

The word arthritis rings alarm bells for many patients when they are first told of the diagnosis. Many patients will be aware of other family members, friends or acquaintances who are very disabled by arthritis and so they look to the future and see themselves in a wheelchair. Although some patients will become very disabled by their OA, the majority will not and it is important to emphasize this. Very often the patient has been worrying about a possible diagnosis of inflammatory arthritis and is greatly relieved to find they have OA. At this initial consultation it is particularly important to emphasize the relatively benign nature of OA, to discuss what patients can do to help themselves in terms of weight loss, exercise, and so on, and to discuss the various treatments available. This kind of counselling, with discussion about joint protection and advice on simple analgesia, may be all that is required initially and we must remember, at this stage, that this person has now become a patient and is asking for professional help.

Because of anxiety, patients often fail to absorb what doctors tell

Table 6.1 Sources of information for patients.

Leaflets and information sheets
Arthritis patient organizations
Meetings
Publications
Recognized websites
Libraries
Videos
Phone helplines

them in consultations and it can be very helpful to give the patient written information to take away. Some arthritis organizations and pharmaceutical companies produce non-promotional booklets and videos on osteoarthritis, which may be of use to some patients. Information may be available on the Internet, for those patients able to access it, although patients should be warned to be selective about the information taken from the worldwide web, as some information may be incorrect or make misleading claims (Table 6.1).

Some patients gain enormous help by joining a patient support group. They may find it helpful to meet fellow sufferers or indeed to realize that others are much worse, or they may become involved in playing an active role in the organization. These people then become an educational resource for their friends. Some patients with OA feel that many of these support groups concentrate almost exclusively on patients with inflammatory joint disease, particularly rheumatoid arthritis, but this approach is changing and OA is becoming recognized as an increasing problem within the community.

Each contact the patient has with a member of the primary care team can potentially provide patient education, not only in OA but also on many other aspects of health and illness. When a patient presents specifically with a problem relating to OA, it is important to use this time to re-take a history and examine the relevant joints and to reinforce advice and counselling. Patients often forget advice they really do not want to hear, such as advice to lose weight or to take more exercise, and they need repeated encouragement to initiate and maintain lifestyle changes. Primary care doctors are usually good at repeating advice and taking a longer term view about education and prevention so that when the patient is ready and the opportunity presents itself, the patient knows they will have the support and encouragement required to make the necessary changes.

Patient education should include the following.

- The nature of OA.
- Strategies for dealing with pain.

- Advice on self-management.
- Written information.
- Support group referral, if appropriate.

Prevention strategies

Education to our patients should also include advice about prevention. Prevention can be divided into three levels.
- Primary prevention, where we try to preserve healthy joints by eliminating risk factors.
- Secondary prevention, by screening for early detection of the disease in possibly asymptomatic individuals and attempting to prevent development of established disease.
- Tertiary prevention, by trying to prevent increasing disability and pain in those who already have established disease.

Primary prevention

As in many disease areas, the aetiology of OA is multifactorial. Some risk factors may be modifiable, others not. One cannot change risk factors of age, sex, family history, congenital abnormality or past trauma, but such patients with one or more risk factors should be targeted for prevention.

Modifiable risk factors for knee and hip OA include obesity, the occurrence of knee injury and jobs requiring bending and carrying. Obesity is an obvious target and ongoing efforts should be made to tackle this growing problem on both an individual and a community basis with increased education in good dietary habits and exercise, leading to healthier lifelong habits (see Chapter 2).

The prevention of knee injury should be tackled by increasing awareness among those participating in sport and their coaches to protect joints by introducing graduated training, warm-up exercises, with stretching, and using joint protection devices, if appropriate.

It would be unrealistic, in our present society, to stop jobs requiring bending and carrying, but increased awareness of the stresses in the joints and the development of techniques to reduce these stresses should be introduced and publicized. In the future, more mechanical or robotic devices should be available to alleviate the problem.

Secondary prevention

At present, although some techniques for detecting early disease in OA are becoming available in an experimental situation, such as specific radiographic techniques, magnetic resonance imaging (MRI) and biochemical markers, we do not yet have the drugs available to prevent the development of progressive or symptomatic disease.

Tertiary prevention

Current knowledge about risk factors affecting progression of pre-existing hip and knee OA is very limited, although at least one study has shown that weight loss decreases pain in knee OA (see Chapter 2). Another study has suggested that dietary factors, and vitamin D in particular, are important in their effect on progressive radiological disease, as opposed to symptomatic disease. Work is also continuing into the potential value of nutritional supplements in the treatment of OA. Gluco-samine and chondroitin sulphate are both simple sugars, which have been shown to have a slow onset symptom modifying effect. Trials are now underway to see whether there is also a structure-modifying effect.

Doctor education

Education into the nature and management of OA for doctors is also imperative. More is being discovered about the nature of OA and there is now some potential for prevention and better management by physical and pharmacological means. It is important that all doctors are aware of these advances and can promote a positive, rather than a negative approach to the condition.

Sources of information for doctors

Information about guidelines, meetings, journals, websites and other educational matters are available from both national and international professional bodies (see Appendix 4).

Behavioural and environmental changes

Behavioural and environmental changes can be proposed for an individual or for the community.

The individual

Looking first at the individual patient with OA, there are a number of lifestyle issues, which a newly diagnosed OA patient should consider.

Body weight

If body weight is normal, the patient should be advised not to let the weight increase. If overweight, advise the patient to lose weight, as there is good evidence that weight loss can reduce pain in knee OA and also reduce progression (see Chapter 2). Maintenance of normal body weight also facilitates exercise and mobility.

Diet

There is no evidence that any specific diet helps OA, but healthy eating will improve the patient's general health and maintain optimal body weight. There is some evidence that dietary and vitamin supplements have an effect on cartilage and progression of OA (see Chapter 2).

Exercise

Certain exercises can be undertaken to improve the musculature around a specific joint, e.g. quadriceps exercises for knee OA. Improvement in muscle strength helps to protect the joint by absorbing extra stresses on the affected joint. General exercise to maintain aerobic fitness is helpful; joints do better if used regularly. Aerobic exercise also helps psychologically by improving general well-being, reducing depression and helping to maintain a healthy weight.

Exercise is good in OA for the following reasons.
- Reduces pain.
- Preserves and restores range of motion.
- Prevents and reduces contractures.
- Preserves joint alignment.
- Maintains proprioception and balance mechanisms.
- May help to reduce depression.
- Helps to maintain normal weight.
- Increases general well-being.

Joint protection

There are some simple lifestyle changes which can provide joint protection. Patients should be told to respect pain from their joints, as pain is a warning sign that there may be a problem and that they may have been over-stressing the joint. Patients should try to move positively and avoid stresses on the joint and uncoordinated loading. They should be advised to spread a heavy workload over a space of time and pace themselves,

6

and to look carefully at the tasks they have to do and try to achieve a balance between activity and rest.

Hobbies

Ask your patients about leisure activities. If a particular aspect of a hobby causes the patient pain, it is much better to consider other approaches, rather than the patient giving up the hobby. For example, if gardening causes the patient with knee OA pain on bending, advise the use of long-handled tools to avoid kneeling or increase ground cover plants to reduce weeding. A specialist occupational therapist may be able to advise about these problems and several companies produce catalogues of aids, which patients can buy.

Home equipment

Patients may ask about home exercise machines. Exercise bicycles and ski trainers may be useful. It may be worthwhile asking a physiotherapist or the local exercise gym trainer for advice on equipment use. A ski machine reduces impact on the knees, while raising fitness and improving arm and leg musculature. Exercise bicycles may not be good for knee OA unless they are correctly adjusted, because the patient may be putting considerable pressure on the knee while it is bent and this can be counterproductive, especially if they have patellofemoral OA.

House adaptations

There are many simple things which patients can organize for themselves to make life easier within the house and to reduce strain on the joints. Use of grab handles, raised toilet seats and handrails on stairs, both in and outdoors can be useful. Patients with knee OA may find the use of a bath difficult as the OA progresses and a shower may often be the answer. Knee OA is the most common cause of a patient having to stop using a bath. Often simple adaptations may be implemented to avoid patients bending or kneeling and again there are a number of pieces of equipment which can simplify daily activities, such as long-handled shoe horns, mats for opening jars, levers on taps and so on.

Patients should always be encouraged to do as much as they can for themselves, whether at home or in residential care and with simple adaptations such as those mentioned above, their independence can be prolonged. Sometimes special equipment, such as a stair lift, is necessary and simpler than moving house.

Behaviour and environmental changes in the community

In many areas there is an increasing awareness of the needs of those members of the community, who have mobility problems, with special needs.

Access to public buildings

Improved access to public buildings, e.g. cinemas, theatres, airports, libraries, etc. These facilities may include ramps, lifts, moving walkways and toilets for the disabled. Things are changing slowly and some countries have specific standards of access to which all public buildings must comply.

Access to health-care facilities

Improved access to health-care facilities, e.g. hospitals, GP surgeries and dental surgeries. Patients may be deterred from coming for advice and help about their OA because of the difficulties of access to simple health care. As well as considering access to the building and moving around within the building, it is also important to remember to provide suitable seating for patients with mobility problems. Such seating should be of a reasonable height to enable patients to sit and stand easily. It is also often helpful if seats have arm rests to help patients push themselves up to a standing position.

Public transport

OA tends to affect the older age group, who can become socially very isolated. Some areas have buses with low walk-on platforms or platforms which descend, as required. Others run dial-a-bus services, where the individual, who is registered with the scheme, can phone for a bus to go to their home.

Social services

- Day centres or lunch clubs, with transport provided, can make an enormous difference to the quality of life of elderly arthritic patients, who would otherwise be confined to their homes.
- Benefits advice—the elderly are often unaware of their entitlement

to benefits and even a little extra money can make a big difference in paying for extra help in the home, transport, e.g. taxis, or such things as extra heating.

• Home helps not only undertake domestic duties but often act as important monitors of the patient's physical and mental health.

Self-help groups

Although doctors do not officially refer patients to self-help groups, it is certainly worth telling patients about these groups and encouraging them to self-refer and to find out more about the innovative arthritis self-management programmes being set up.

Behaviour decisions of patients and doctors

Patient's decisions

People in the community with musculoskeletal problems are continually making conscious and subconscious decisions about whether or not to seek help. These decisions are determined by the characteristics and belief of the person and such things as the social and cultural environment. People's expectations change because of medical advances (surgical and pharmacological), social changes, media publicity and political and policy decisions.

It is considered that up to 40% of patients with OA do not seek help, even though OA causes pain, even severe pain. We also know that not all our patients wish to take tablets, or a particular class of drugs, such as non-steroidal anti-inflammatory agents. Listed below are some of the possible reasons that people with arthritis do not consult their doctor.

Possible barriers to consultation with a GP

• Belief that joint pain is a part of normal ageing.
• Resignation to pain and disability.
• Fear of painful examination and investigation.
• High prevalence of negative attitudes to OA and arthroplasty (especially total knee replacement).
• Previous unsatisfactory experiences with the medical profession.
• Previous unsatisfactory experiences of relatives and friends.
• Messages that 'nothing can be done' from the medical profession.
• Plausible options offered by alternative practitioners.

In most health-care systems, the majority of patients only have access to a surgeon through a primary care doctor. We therefore need to look at what factors may affect referral. Some people, for instance, are very uncertain about operations.

The public's perception of joint replacement surgery varies markedly between the two major procedures. Total hip arthroplasty is deemed to be a highly successful operation, whereas total knee arthroplasty is still perceived to be in development with not such a good outcome. As primary care changes, so will barriers to consultation with a GP. As GPs are in contact with the general public in many guises, it is important that we continue to inform and advise and try to dispel some of the myths summarized in 'possible barriers to consultation with a GP'.

Doctor's decisions

Factors affecting referral from primary care to an orthopaedic surgeon

- Primary care doctor's ability to diagnose and assess severity early.
- Experience and interests of the primary care doctor.
- Severity of the problem.
- Attitudes of the primary care doctor to orthopaedic surgery.
- Relationship of primary care doctor to local surgeons.
- Access to surgery.
- Access to alternatives, including physical therapy.
- Presence or absence of referral guidelines.
- Costs.

A doctor's training is a life-long experience and we need continually to reassess and appraise our educational needs. This way we will remain open minded and more likely to accept changes and new ideas.

The flow diagram of OA patients pathways (Fig. 6.1) shows the routes which people may take when seeking or not seeking medical help and advice. Some people never seek formal medical help, be they symptomatic or asymptomatic (point A on the diagram). Some people stop seeking help at various stages throughout their management. Perhaps they think that conventional medicine has nothing to offer them. This is the patient's choice and we should respect these wishes.

Often we do not know why patients fail to return or choose to return after a long absence. It is important, however, that patients know that a primary care doctor is always available when patients choose to seek help. The flow diagram shows the pathways but does not suggest reasons for individual choices or actions.

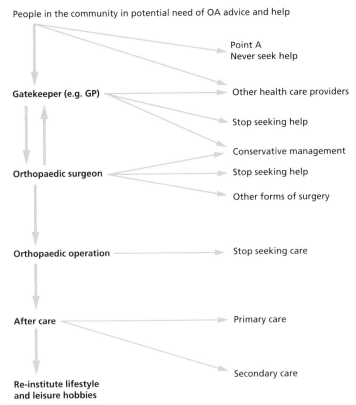

People in the community in potential need of OA advice and help

Point A
Never seek help

Gatekeeper (e.g. GP)

Other health care providers

Stop seeking help

Conservative management

Orthopaedic surgeon

Stop seeking help

Other forms of surgery

Orthopaedic operation

Stop seeking care

After care

Primary care

Secondary care

Re-institute lifestyle
and leisure hobbies

Fig. 6.1 Flow diagram of patient pathways. Adapted from [1] with permission.

Management—the way forward

The increasing realization of the impact of chronic non-life-threatening disease on the health of people is changing priorities and increasing emphasis is being placed on ways of decreasing this morbidity within the community. New ways of developing care are becoming apparent with the setting up of community priorities involving both primary and secondary care, with a change in standard referral patterns and increasing involvement of other health professionals. The primary care team for patients with rheumatic conditions might include nursing staff, both practice and community based, physiotherapists, occupational therapists, dieticians, chiropodists/podiatrists and social services personnel to offer help with day care, home helps, bath attendants and benefits and so on. All members of the team should be able to work together to give the greatest benefit to these community-based patients, under the overall coordinating care of the GP. The concept of clinical governance will also provide standards based on peer review and should gradually improve the management of patients with chronic OA in the community.

Audit

Having set various standards, it is up to all of us working in the field to implement audit projects to examine whether we are meeting standards and continuing to show improvement in management. Audit in OA is often difficult. Some of the recognized measures for testing pain and disability, such as the WOMAC scale or Lequesne indices are time con-suming to apply routinely in primary care and as OA is a condition with periods of stability, often dispersed with acute flares, such indices (see Appendix 2), if only applied occasionally, may give a false picture. Drug therapy can be audited but it is important to remember to include over-the-counter drugs, as well as prescription drugs, otherwise again a false picture will emerge. Perhaps more emphasis should be placed on tackling obesity and trying to help patients to lose weight and attain and maintain a normal body weight, and to increase exercise. Audits to assess these could be set up.

Common questions and answers

1 Question: Is OA hereditary?

   Answer: There is a form of OA, nodal OA, which is associated with a particular gene (*HLA-A1 B8* gene). This may be associated with OA occurring at a younger than usual age group and is more common in the daughters of affected patients.

2 Question: Will OA affect all my joints?

   Answer: OA tends to affect knees, hands, hips and spine, and less com-monly wrists, shoulders, toes and ankles. Some patients can develop generalized OA affecting several joints but many patients will have only one or two joints affected.

3 Question: Will it help my knee OA if I lose weight?

   Answer: Yes, there is good evidence that weight loss in patients who are overweight will considerably reduce the pain from OA knee.

4 Question: Will HRT help my joint pain?

   Answer: HRT often increases general well-being and so increases activ-ity, which may in itself help the symptoms of OA. There is also some evid-ence that HRT may decrease the risk of developing OA of the hip and knee.

5 Question: Will a vegetarian diet help my OA?

   Answer: There is no evidence that a vegetarian diet helps OA. There is, however, a little evidence that good nutrition, in particular with vitamins C and D, can prevent progression of OA and some simple sugars, such as chondroitin and glucosamine may have a slow symptom-modifying effect.

6 Question: Does my OA mean I must stop my daily walking?

Answer: No, it is very important that you continue to take sensible exercise on a regular basis to keep the muscles around the joints in good condition. Joints are meant to be used.

7 Question: When my joint hurts, will I damage it if I use it?

Answer: For the normal background pain of OA, it is better to take regular simple analgesics and move the joint. This will not cause damage but will improve the condition by improving the muscles around the joint. If your joint becomes inflamed or swollen, it is sensible to rest it until the acute inflammatory flare settles before resuming normal exercise.

8 Question: Does living in a damp climate cause OA?

Answer: There is no evidence that living in a damp climate actually causes OA, but there does seem to be a relationship between joint pain and damp weather, and patients often complain that their joints ache more in damp weather.

9 Question: Now I have OA, can I get rid of it?

Answer: OA is a dynamic condition and repair of damage is always taking place. Many people only experience intermittent problems and have long spells with only mild symptoms or indeed no symptoms at all.

10 Question: Is swimming good for knee OA?

Answer: The kick of breaststroke puts lateral pressure on the knee, which can exacerbate knee OA. Swimming itself is good exercise and so you can continue swimming using backstroke or crawl, where the leg movement is less stressful to the knee joint.

Reference

1 Dieppe P, Basler H-D, Chard P et al. Knee replacement study for osteoarthritis: effectiveness, practice variations, indications and possible determinants of utilization. Rheumatology 1999; 38: 73–83.

CHAPTER 7

Physical Therapy and Mechanical Interventions

Physical therapy has an important role in the management of osteo-arthritis (OA), although there is limited objective evidence of the benefits of such treatments. It is often difficult to undertake controlled and/or randomized clinical trials in physiotherapy because of the nature of the interventions and the obvious difficulty of blinding patients and investigators. One study on patients with knee OA, using a control group, has shown the benefit of an exercise regime on quadriceps function and disability, with maintenance of improvement at 6 months [1]. Such therapy, however, is expensive in therapist's time to teach and supervise exercise programmes and ensure long-term compliance by some form of follow-up. Conversely, such therapy may reduce the need for expensive and potentially hazardous interventions, such as drug therapy and surgery.

Physical management includes the following.
- Physiotherapy.
- Aids and appliances.
- Impact-absorbing footwear.

Physiotherapy

The first aim of physiotherapy is education and advice. This should include advice on the following.
- Rest and exercise.
- Pacing activities.
- Posture, if appropriate.
- Joint protection and how to decrease stress on affected joints.
- Building up specific muscle groups, with demonstration of specific exercises and encouragement to keep this up on a long-term basis (Fig. 7.1).

One limiting factor in the effectiveness of physiotherapy is getting over to patients the importance of their own physical involvement in the treatment. Many patients still expect physiotherapists to apply interventions and do things to them, rather than the patient taking an active role in their own therapy. Changing a patient's attitudes is often a difficult and time-consuming task.

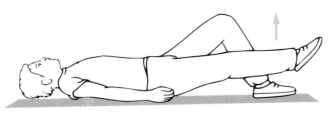

Straight-leg raise — lying
Hold for slow count of 5
Repeat 5 times each leg

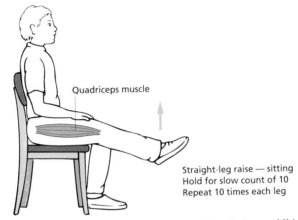

Quadriceps muscle

Straight-leg raise — sitting
Hold for slow count of 10
Repeat 10 times each leg

Fig. 7.1 Quadriceps exercise. From the Primary Care Rheumatology Society and Shire Pharmaceuticals with permission.

Other key aims of physiotherapy are as follows.

- To decrease pain.
- To increase mobility.
- To help to restore function.
- To limit disease progression.
- To prevent long-term problems.

Thermal treatments

In OA, heat is more often used than cold, but cold may be worth trying especially to relieve pain during postoperative rehabilitation. Heat may help to increase the range of movements and decrease joint contractures. Heat can be used as superficial heat, with hot packs or pads, or as deep heat with therapeutic ultrasound or short-wave or microwave diathermy. Hot baths or showers may ease pain in large joints after exercise.

Transcutaneous electrical nerve stimulation (TENS)

This is a battery-operated device that generates an electrical waveform and transmits it via electrode pads to the skin. The rationale for this therapy depends on the gate theory of pain. TENS produces a stimulus in the larger fibres, which then pass through the gate rendering it closed to smaller fibres, which would normally transmit the pain sensation to the higher centres. TENS can produce different pulse widths and also variable rates of stimulation and patients should experiment to find what suits them best. For most patients a frequency in the range of 50–100 Hz is the most effective and this produces a comfortable tingling sensation. Not only can TENS produce a degree of analgesia in some patients, it may give sufficient relief to allow stiff and painful muscles to be put through a greater range of movement and therefore gradually improve the basic condition. Some patients find TENS of no value at all, whereas others may experience prolonged relief. Pain clinics and physiotherapy departments often lend TENS machines out and, in some instances, patients buy them directly from the suppliers. It is always worth asking advice on which to buy from your local physiotherapy department. Their advice usually produces large cost savings for the patient.

Hydrotherapy

Some patients find hydrotherapy of great value but it is an expensive form of therapy and only available in certain centres. Some patients undertake almost their own form of hydrotherapy by taking part in water aerobic sessions held at many leisure centres or performing their own exercise regime after a hot bath.

Physical measures—taping and splinting

This might include patellar taping (Fig. 7.2) for knee OA. This may be a useful treatment for patellofemoral knee OA. The patella is taped medially and the alteration of the alignment of the patella may give pain relief [2].

OA of the first carpometacarpal joint at the thumb is often helped by provision of a resting splint (Fig. 7.3, p. 82).

Knee braces, which fit around the thigh and around the upper calf, and are attached by sophisticated hinge mechanisms, may be useful and may help to correct abnormal biomechanics, especially in unstable knees (Fig. 7.4, p. 82).

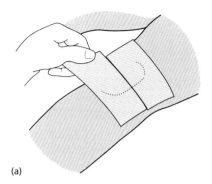

Tape the knee with two pieces of
stretch tape so that the
patella is completely covered.
Do not put on under tension.

(a)

7

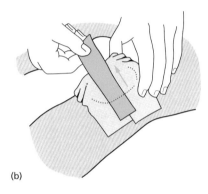

If glide of patella needs correcting,
apply tensioning tape at the lateral
patella border medially, lift soft tissue
towards the midline and affix tape at the
medial femoral condyle.

(b)

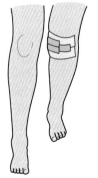

After taping, repeat the activity which
previously caused the pain. If the pain is
not considerably reduced the taping
may be incorrectly applied or a different
taping technique may be required.

(c)

Fig. 7.2 Patella taping to treat patellofemoral pain. From Biersdorf with permission.

Adaptive aids

Ask the patient what tasks or activities he or she is finding difficult.
Some companies produce brochures of aids for all sorts of purposes. An
occupational therapist is the best person to advise patients on aids

7

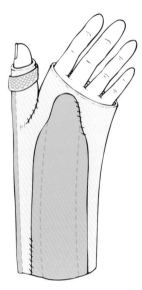

Fig. 7.3 A resting thumb splint.

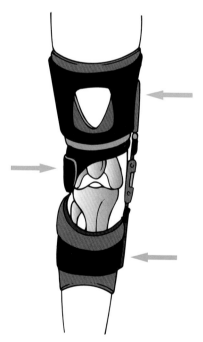

Fig. 7.4 A knee brace.

and appliances for specific needs. Access to occupational therapy may be through community referral or through a hospital outpatient department.
• *Environmental aids*, e.g. rails, handles, stairlifts, ramps, key holders, doorknob extensions, etc.

- *Walking aids*, e.g. sticks, tripods and wheeled aids.
- *Transport aids*, e.g. wheelchairs.
- *Transfer aids.* These help to transfer patients from sitting to standing, as many patients can manage to walk once they are in the upright position but cannot raise themselves without help. Transfer aids include higher seats, armrests and spring-loaded or power-lift armchairs.
- *Toilet aids*, e.g. raised toilet seat, toilet frame.
- *Bathing aids*, e.g. seats, non-slip mats, hoists.
- *Personal hygiene aids*, e.g. long-handled brushes, long-handled toothbrushes and tap levers.
- *Dressing aids*, e.g. buttonhooks, long-handled shoehorns, stocking aids, using Velcro instead of buttons.
- *Feeding aids*, e.g. two-handled cup, large-handled cutlery, easily opened lids on medication.
- *Recreational aids*, e.g. book holders, remote controls for televisions and other appliances. There are also some specialist aids for recreational activities, such as fishing, bowling, snooker and gardening.
- *Communication aids*, e.g. pre-set numbers, speaker phones, remote control door opener.
- *Housework aids*, e.g. long-handled instruments, potholders, and the use of machines, e.g. blenders and food processors, electric can openers, use of sponge rather than cloths.

Some of these adaptive aids are shown in Fig. 7.5.

Footwear

It seems logical that the impact of a heel striking a concrete pavement would produce jarring in the joints above the point of impact and could irritate joints already affected by OA, especially hip and knee. The ankle is rarely involved in OA. The use of some impact-absorbing footwear can reduce this stress on the joint. Impact-absorbing footwear can be as simple as a good training shoe or alternatively an impact-absorbing insole, which can often be bought in sports shops, can be placed in the patient's own shoes.

Features of shoes suitable for lower limb osteoarthritis

- Flat shoe.
- Soft impact-absorbing sole.
- Broad forefoot.
- Soft upper.

Sometimes a lateral wedge, placed in the patient's shoe, can relieve pain

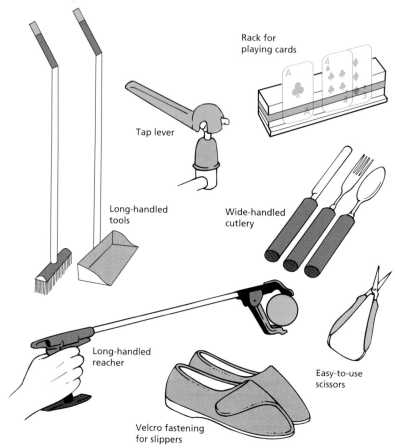

Rack for playing cards

Tap lever

Long-handled tools

Wide-handled cutlery

Long-handled reacher

Easy-to-use scissors

Velcro fastening for slippers

Fig. 7.5 Adaptive aids: poor grip can be helped by enlarging handles and extending levers, whilst difficult reaching can be overcome by using longer handles.

of lower limb OA by correcting a varus deformity. It is a simple strategy well worth trying, as it may give considerable benefit. If not, the patient will soon stop using it!

References

1   Hurley MV, Scott DL. Improvements in quadriceps sensorimotor function and disability of patients with knee osteoarthritis following a clinically practicable exercise regime. *Br J Rheumatol* 1998; 37: 1181–7.
2   Cushnaghan J, MacCarthy C, Dieppe P. Taping the patella medially; a new treatment for OA of the knee joint? *BMJ* 1994; 308: 753–5.

CHAPTER 8

Pharmacological Treatment

Our main aims in drug therapy are to relieve pain, decreasing but not necessarily eliminating pain, and to minimize risk to patients.

It is good practice to start drug therapy with the simplest and safest agents, paracetamol should therefore be the first choice before progressing on to more potent and potentially more risky agents if and when required (Table 8.1).

Many of these drug therapies can be used in combination, but not all. See Table 8.2 for some practical considerations.

Table 8.1 Suggested order for drug therapy.	
	Paracetamol
	Topical preparations
	topical non-steroid anti-inflammatory drugs (NSAIDs)
	capsaicin
	Compound analgesics or ibuprofen
	Ibuprofen plus analgesics
	Other oral NSAIDs
	Other oral NSAIDs plus analgesics
	Steroid injection
	Intra-articular hyaluronan
	Tricyclic antidepressant—may be considered at any stage in the above order

Table 8.2 Drug combinations—practical points.	
	Capsaicin may be used with oral analgesics and NSAIDs
	Topical NSAIDs may be used with oral analgesics
	Oral NSAIDs may be used with analgesics but do not give two NSAIDs together
	Steroid injection and intra-articular hyaluronan may be used with oral NSAIDs and/or analgesics
	Amitriptyline may be used with all the above therapies

Paracetamol

Many patients require much education to take paracetamol seriously. They think of it either as very dangerous, because of publicity regarding overdosage or ineffective as they can buy it in the supermarket and it can take a great deal of time to encourage patients to realize that paracetamol is both safe and effective. Patients often fail to take adequate dosage and 1 g four times a day may be needed to give adequate pain relief. Paracetamol has few side-effects and few interactions, although it may interfere with warfarin and should not be given with metoclopramide. Its main disadvantage is that it has to be taken regularly, every 4–6 h.

Many patients will get good results from this regime but some may require additional or alternative therapy if they have increasing pain or sustain an inflammatory flare.

Topical preparations

Topical preparations should be considered as the next choice and can be particularly helpful in OA of the knee or the small joints of the hand and in the elbow, wrist and ankle. It has been argued that the benefits of all topical preparations are due to the process of rubbing itself, acting as massage. There are, however, many studies which show a benefit of using a topical agent over placebo, where both are being rubbed on. Another benefit of a topical agent, which is sometimes disregarded, is that all topical therapies give patients a degree of control over their own condition, and psychologically this may be extremely valuable. Three groups of topical preparations are available.

Rubs or embrocations

These products appear to work by producing counterirritation of the skin, which stimulates the sensory nerves, which then compete with the pain signals produced by the affected area, resulting in a decrease in the pain message transmitted to the brain from the affected area.

Some preparations contain rubefacients, such as capsicum, salicylates and nicontinates, which give a feeling of warmth and vasodilatation, while others contain camphor or menthol, which give a sensation of coolness. These products have been available for many years and there is little evidence to support their usage but some patients find them helpful and they are very safe. They can be used in conjunction with oral analgesics.

Topical non-steroidal anti-inflammatory drugs

These preparations contain NSAIDs in a form suitable for rubbing over the affected joint. For a long time these preparations have been considered by many doctors to be ineffective and expensive and are not included in many formularies. It has been shown, however, that therapeutic levels of the active drug can be found in the synovial fluid and surrounding tissues after use but without the high serum levels obtained after an oral dose of the drug, thus reducing systemic side-effects.

A recent meta-analysis [1] has shown that topical NSAIDs can be effective in many acute and chronic conditions, including OA, and around 1 in 3 patients achieve 50% reduction in pain over and above the effect of placebo.

Although side-effects of topical NSAIDs are not common, they should still not be prescribed to patients who have a contraindication to oral NSAID therapy, as there is some systemic absorption.

Capsaicin

This is a topical cream made from hot chillies. It is said to act by depleting substance P, which is a neuropeptide involved in the transmission of pain in the afferent nerve fibres. Substance P levels are raised in inflamed joints and substance P is also thought to stimulate synoviocytes to produce prostaglandins and collagenases. The rationale of treatment with 0.25% capsaicin cream is that by gradually reducing the levels of substance P within the joint, less pain is transmitted to the higher centres. Studies have shown a successive decrease in OA pain, with the maximum benefit experienced after around 4 weeks of therapy. Capsaicin cream has to be applied four times a day, as a very small bead. The main disadvantages are stinging or burning sensations experienced by around 46% of patients. In clinical practice most patients improve over the first few weeks of treatment. Care must also be taken to wash hands immediately after application to avoid contact with sensitive body areas, such as the eyes.

Capsaicin has been used in the USA for over 10 years and is suggested by the American College of Rheumatology guidelines for the management of knee OA as the next stage in pharmacological therapy, following paracetamol.

Compound analgesics

If paracetamol and topical therapies are not effective, the next stage might be a compound analgesic. There are a number of analgesic preparations available over the counter from pharmacies and when prescribing for a patient, it is really important to find out what, if anything, they are buying from the pharmacist to avoid problems of overdosage or interaction. It is also important to ask the patient about dosage, as you may frequently find that they take more than the recommended dose.

Psychologically if you prescribe a weaker analgesic than the one already being taken, the patient may lose confidence. Paracetamol and codeine combinations are the most common of the compound analgesics. There are also various combinations of paracetamol and codeine together with caffeine, codeine and aspirin, and paracetamol and dihydrocodeine, in various strengths. Some of these are available over the counter while others are only available as prescription medicines.

Coproxamol, a compound opiate containing paracetamol 325 mg plus dextropropoxyphene is widely prescribed and many patients find it effective, although central nervous system (CNS) side-effects can occur and dependence may develop.

There is no specific hierarchy for use of the preparations, as patients have an individual response to the various ingredients, but it is logical to start at as low a dose as possible and increase the strength of preparations if and when required.

The Oxford Pain Site [2] have advocated a three-pot system for patients with chronic osteoarthritic pain. They have divided these patients into two groups, those who can and those who cannot take NSAIDs.

- For those who can take NSAIDs:
    for mild pain—2 paracetamol;
    for moderate pain—2 Co-codamol *or* 1 ibuprofen;
    for severe pain—2 Co-codamol *and* 1 ibuprofen.
- For those who cannot take NSAIDs:
    for mild pain—2 paracetamol;
    for moderate pain—1 Co-codamol and 1 paracetamol;
    for severe pain—2 Co-codamol.

The pain of OA may vary considerably from day to day, and this system is sufficiently flexible to allow patients the freedom to decide which particular drug regime they choose to use on a daily basis.

Stronger analgesics

Some patients with severe OA, especially of the lower limb, may require stronger analgesics. These can often be effective but their use may be limited by side-effects.
- Strong paracetamol/codeine combinations are effective but may give CNS side-effects and constipation, e.g. paracetamol 500 mg plus codeine phosphate 30 mg.
- Codeine by itself is very constipating and not often used.
- Dihydrocodeine also causes constipation and can give nausea, vomiting and CNS side-effects. It is an effective analgesic but may be addictive.

- Meptazinol is an opiate partial agonist, said to have a low incidence of respiratory depression but can cause nausea and vomiting.
- Tramadol is an opiate analogue, with two mechanisms of action. It has an opiate effect and also enhances serotoninergic and adrenergic pathways and in theory gives fewer opioid side-effects but can cause some psychiatric reactions.
- Nefopam (Acupan) is a non-opioid preparation, chemically a benzox-azocine. It can be effective in a number of patients but can give sympathetic and antimuscarinic side-effects.

Antidepressants

Tricyclic antidepressant drugs can have a role in improving pain relief, when given in low doses together with analgesics. These drugs are known to be effective in neurogenic pain and may act by modifying the pain response. They may also have an antidepressant effect, which can be particularly useful in patients with chronic pain and they can relieve disturbed sleep when given in the evening or at bedtime. A low dose of 10 mg to start may be effective, although some patients will need increments to 25 or 50 mg at night. If tricyclics are not effective, one of the SSRI (selective serotonin receptor inhibitors) may be useful at low dose. Remember that depression itself may be common in severe OA and may need treatment with antidepressants at full therapeutic dose.

Non-steroidal anti-inflammatory drugs

NSAIDs have both an analgesic and anti-inflammatory effect. Until recently it was thought that there was no inflammation in OA but this view is changing, and most OA joints probably do have some mild inflammatory changes. Many OA joints will experience flares of inflammation from time to time and on these occasions the inflammatory signs may be obvious. This low-grade inflammation in joints may be the reason why some patients respond well to NSAID therapy, while others do equally well with simple analgesics.

From a practical point of view NSAIDs are probably over prescribed. Patients like these drugs, as they often seem to give better symptom control than analgesics. In particular, NSAIDs are very effective where stiffness is a problem, and dosage regimes are usually simpler than for analgesics.

One study [3] looked at a group of patients with knee OA, who were already on an NSAID. This group of patients was randomized into a placebo group or a diclofenac group, with paracetamol as escape

medication, and the patients were followed up over 2 years. Some patients suffered a flare in their symptoms on discontinuing NSAID and this
subgroup did seem to require NSAID therapy. Another group, however,
coped for 2 years without an NSAID, having previously been established
on this therapy, suggesting that many patients do not actually require
NSAID treatment. Some patients seem to feel very much better, and
have better pain control, on certain NSAIDs than others. Many patients
have worked out for themselves the best way of taking NSAIDs and take
them as required, perhaps reserving them for times when they know
that they are going to be undertaking extra activity.

Mode of action

In 1971 Sir John Vane proposed the theory that NSAIDs work by inhibiting the biosynthesis of prostaglandins, which lead to the development of
inflammation. It was eventually found that NSAIDs were inhibiting the
enzyme cyclo-oxygenase (COX), which was leading to the production of
prostaglandins.

In 1991 two isoforms of COX were discovered (Fig. 8.1).
• COX 1 is the constitutive (or housekeeping) form which, when
activated, leads to the production of prostacyclin (which protects the
gastric mucosa), prostaglandin E_2 (which protects kidney function) and
thromboxane A (which protects platelet function).
• COX 2 is the inducible (or inflammatory) form which, when activated, leads to the production of proteases, prostaglandins and other
inflammatory mediators leading to inflammation.

Classical NSAIDs block both COX 1 and 2 activity, so while they are
effective in decreasing inflammation, they may lead to the loss of gastric
and renal protection.

In theory an ideal NSAID would be one which blocked the development of inflammation while preserving gastric protection and renal
function.

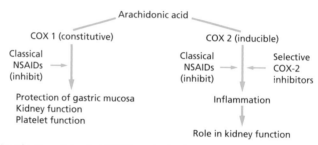

Fig. 8.1 Site of action of classical NSAIDs and selective COX 2 inhibitors.

Limitations to NSAID use

The main limiting factors to the use of oral NSAIDs are the contraindications, interactions and the risk of side-effects.

Side-effects

Side-effects can be very serious in terms of gastrointestinal bleeding, ulceration or perforation, and although numbers of such side-effects are fairly high across the country, most GPs have only rarely encountered such problems in their own patients. The often dramatic presentation of gastric problems perhaps overshadows the more insidious but potentially equally serious side-effects of renal damage.

These drugs can cause dyspepsia, nausea, diarrhoea, peptic ulceration and acute gastrointestinal bleeding, which may be catastrophic or chronic gastrointestinal bleeding, leading to anaemia. They can cause fluid retention and may precipitate congestive cardiac failure. They can lead to renal failure, especially in patients with pre-existing renal impairment and can, rarely, cause interstitial fibrosis or papillary necrosis. They can cause hypersensitivity reactions such as bronchospasm, skin rash and angio-oedema and can precipitate or exacerbate colitis. In some patients NSAIDs cause CNS side-effects, such as tinnitus, photosensitivity, headache and personality change.

Classical NSAIDs—gastric side-effects

Following some comparative studies of the side-effects of NSAIDs, the Committee for Safety of Medicines (UK) in 1994 advised on the relative safety of seven NSAIDs with regard to serious upper gastrointestinal side-effects (Table 8.3). The newer NSAIDs and COX 2 inhibitors were not included at the time of this report.

Table 8.3 Relative risks of NSAIDs with regard to serious upper gastrointestinal side-effects.

Lowest risk	Ibuprofen
Intermediate risk	Diclofenac
	Indomethacin
	Naproxen
	Ketoprofen
	Piroxicam (at higher end of intermediate group)
High risk	Azapropazone

Contraindications to NSAID use

- Active peptic ulceration.
- Pregnancy and lactation.
- Haemophilia.
- Aspirin or NSAID allergy.
- Angioneurotic oedema.

Relative contraindications

Cases where NSAIDs may be used if necessary, with special care.
- Past history of peptic ulceration or gastrointestinal bleed.
- Current dyspepsia.
- Asthma.
- Renal impairment.
- Congestive cardiac failure.
- Hypertension.
- Hepatic impairment.
- Warfarin therapy.

Interactions

NSAIDs may interact with many other drugs. Some interactions apply to all NSAIDs (class effect), while others may be specific for a particular drug. The main class interactions are with anticoagulants, diuretics, lithium, methotrexate, quinolone antibiotics, oral hypoglycaemics, angiotensin-converting enzyme (ACE) inhibitors and β-blockers. Some NSAIDs may also interact with cyclosporin, hydantoins and digoxin.

Special precautions

The elderly, especially females, smokers and those on long-term steroids are at highest risk of developing complications of NSAID therapy. Elderly patients are more likely to suffer from other medical conditions where NSAIDs may cause problems, such as renal failure, or they may be taking other drugs, such as antihypertensives or digoxin, giving the potential for interactions. Elderly patients, however, are those most likely to have more severe OA and perhaps be more likely to be considered for NSAID treatment. If NSAIDs are thought to be necessary for an acute inflammatory flare or failure to control pain by any other measures, they should be prescribed at the lowest dose and for the shortest time possible. Care should be taken when NSAIDs are put onto

8

a computerized repeat prescribing system, as these drugs can then be given out on a regular basis with no monitoring, either of side-effects or of the need for continuing prescription.

Co-prescription

If a patient at high risk of gastric side-effects requires an NSAID, the co-prescription of misoprostol, to prevent gastric and duodenal ulceration, or ranitidine, to prevent duodenal ulceration may be required. The use of misoprostol has shown a 40% relative reduction in serious gastrointestinal events but it may cause indigestion and diarrhoea. Routine co-prescription of misoprostol has not been shown to be cost-effective. Proton pump inhibitors are also licensed for the treatment and prophylaxis of NSAID ulceration.

Selective COX 2 inhibitors

Several NSAIDs have some selective COX 2 inhibition. Those available at present are etodolac, meloxicam and nabumetone, all of which seem to have fewer gastric side-effects than other classical NSAIDs.

Coxibs or COX 2 specific inhibitors

Coxibs, pharmaceutical agents which specifically block COX 2, have recently been developed. Coxibs leave intact COX 1 thus preserving gastric protection, while blocking COX 2 thus blocking inflammation. Both COX 1 and COX 2 seem to have a constitutive role which is important in maintaining renal function and it is not yet clear whether the renal side-effects of coxibs will differ from that of non-selective NSAIDs. Two of these compounds, rofecoxib and celecoxib, are more than 100 times as selective in their ability to block COX 2 as the currently available NSAIDs, and appear to have a similar profile to placebo in their propensity to cause gastroduodenal ulceration [4]. If they live up to this promise when used widely in the community, these drugs should provide safer drug treatment for the management of the pain and stiffness of OA.

Intra-articular steroids

Patients with an acute inflammatory flare of OA or acute crystal-related synovitis may benefit greatly from an intra-articular steroid injection. The effect of such an injection usually lasts around 4–5 weeks, by which time the inflammatory flare has often settled. Some patients, however, derive great benefit from an intra-articular injection and the effect may last for several months. Some patients with moderate to severe OA request an injection before putting some additional stress on their joints, such as going on holiday or attending a wedding, and this can greatly relieve symptoms in the short term.

Some patients, while awaiting surgery for OA knee, benefit from an injection but technically this can be difficult as the bony contours are abnormal and often there is hardly any joint space remaining. Others in a similar situation find no benefit from a steroid injection, as the joint destruction is too great for the steroid to have any effect. Current practice suggests there should be an interval of 4 weeks between injections given into a specific joint up to a maximum of four injections in 1 year, although two or three different joints can be injected at the same time.

Contraindications

- Joint infection—If you think that the joint may be infected, do not inject steroid. Send any aspirated synovial fluid for culture.
- Local skin infection near to the injection site.
- Systemic infection.
- Hypersensitivity to any ingredient in the injection, including the local anaesthetic.
- First 16 weeks of pregnancy.
- Diabetes, hypertension, osteoporosis and hypothyroidism are relative contraindications to steroid injection.

Side-effects

Side-effects to steroid injections are not common but the following may occur.
- Transient flare of inflammation and pain.
- Septic arthritis.
- Hypersensitivity reaction.
- Localized subcutaneous fat atrophy.
- Transient hyperglycaemia.
- Tendon rupture.
- Aseptic osteonecrosis.
- Flushing.
- Delay of menstruation.
- Post menopausal bleeding.

Table 8.4 Steroid dosages for different joints.		
Knee	1 ml
CMC joint	Up to 0.5 ml
AC joint	0.2–0.5 ml
Shoulder	1 ml steroid plus 1–10 ml of 1% lidocaine, if appropriate
Trochanteric bursitis	1 ml

Preparations of intra-articular steroids

There are three commonly used intra-articular preparations.
- Hydrocortisone acetate 25 mg/ml (Hydrocortistab).
- Methylprednisolone acetate 40 mg/ml (Depo-Medrone).
- Triamcinolone hexacetonide 20 mg/ml (Lederspan).

Hydrocortisone acetate is shorter acting and less potent, and is probably used more for soft tissue problems than intra-articular injections. Methylprednisolone is medium acting and of moderate potency, while triamcinolone is longer acting and the most potent of the three. If required, local anaesthetic can be used to infiltrate the area of injection. This, however, sometimes obscures the landmarks and makes the injection technically more difficult. Many doctors prefer either to mix local anaesthetic with the steroid preparation (both hydrocortisone acetate and triamcinolone hexacetonide have a licence allowing this) or to use a pre-mixed preparation, such as Depo-Medrone with lidocaine, which is methylprednisolone acetate 40 mg/ml plus lidocaine 10 mg/ml. Suitable volumes for different joints are shown in Table 8.4.

Intra-articular hyaluronans

In a normal joint, hyaluronic acid provides the synovial fluid with its viscoelastic properties, which are essential for shock absorption and lubrication. Hyaluronic acid also seems to have a role in joint repair and possibly also to have some anti-inflammatory and analgesic action.

Clinical trials have suggested that a series of hyaluronan injections can alleviate the pain and stiffness of knee OA for up to 6 months and have shown comparable or slightly better results than daily NSAIDs, but with fewer side-effects. These products can, however, give some local reactions of pain and swelling.

Two preparations are available.
- Hyaluronic acid 20 mg/2 ml: this is given as a series of once weekly injections for 5 weeks.
- Hylan GF20 16 mg/2 ml: given as a series of once weekly injections for 3 weeks.

One study with hyaluronic acid compared with triamcinolone hexacetonide showed similar short-term efficacy but the patients in the hyaluronic acid group had significantly less pain at 6 months. Further studies are awaited to determine whether or not the use of these compounds has an impact on surgical referrals.

Future drug therapy

A number of biological agents have been found to have potentially beneficial properties in arthritis but they present a difficult challenge in delivery into the appropriate place, and at the appropriate stage, of the OA process. Techniques are being developed, using gene transfer to aid delivery of these agents into joints and other tissues. These agents could then target very specific areas and hopefully give more prolonged benefit, with fewer side-effects.

The degenerative changes seen in OA are thought to result from an imbalance between catabolic and anabolic processes. The catabolic processes are induced by the cytokines, interleukin 1 (IL-1) and tumour necrosing factor (TNF). Inhibition of the activity of these cytokines may block cartilage breakdown. Diacerrhein is a new compound, which is undergoing clinical trials at present. Diacerrhein antagonizes IL-1 and may act as a disease-modifying drug for OA.

Recent research has shown that nitric oxide plays a role in the pathophysiology of OA and controlling nitric oxide production might have a potentially beneficial effect. There has also been considerable research into inhibiting matrix metalloprotease (MMP) activity as a treatment for arthritis and antibiotics such as tetracycline and its semisynthetic forms doxycycline and minocycline show significant properties of inhibition against MMP activity.

If may be some time before these agents are available for use in the routine clinical situation but the prospects for impacting on OA look very promising.

Summary points

- Simple analgesia, in adequate dose, should be used first. Encourage patients to take full dosage (4 g) of paracetamol on bad days.
- Safe topical therapies may assist pain relief.
- NSAIDs may be helpful in some patients but should be used with care.
- Low dose tricyclic antidepressants may be useful.
- Intra-articular steroid injections may be used for acute flares.
- Intra-articular hyaluronan injection may alleviate pain and stiffness in knee OA.
- Newer COX 2 specific blockers may reduce serious side-effects.

8

References

1 Moore RA, Tramer MR, Caroll D *et al.* Quantitative systematic review of topically applied non-steroidal anti-inflammatory drugs. *BMJ* 1998; 316: 333–8.
2 Oxford Pain Research Website: http://www.ebando.com
3 Dieppe P, Cushnaghan J, Jasani MK, McCrae F, Watts I. A two year, placebo controlled trial of non-steroidal anti-inflammatory therapy in osteoarthritis of the knee joint. *Br J Rheumatol* 1993; 32: 595–600.
4 Wolfe MM, Lichtenstein DR, Singh G. Gastrointestinal toxicity of nonsteroidal antiinflammatory drugs. *N Engl J Med* 1999; 340 (24): 1888–99.

CHAPTER 9

Surgical Options and Procedures

Patients often require information from primary care doctors concerning surgical treatments or procedures. Osteoarthritis (OA) is a dynamic process, which suggests that we can influence the process. Age and the person's activity levels both influence the individual's treatment and surgical choices.

In this chapter, we will consider procedures that may influence and possibly limit progression, as well as operations to treat the disability and pain caused by advanced disease. We will discuss which patients will most benefit from treatment, and the use of referral forms, preferably developed locally. Today, with the trend towards shorter hospital stays and day surgery, postoperative rehabilitation and information for the primary care teams, patients and their carers is most important.

Some surgical procedures such as arthroscopy may be undertaken by primary care doctors who have a particular knowledge and interest in OA and rheumatology. Other practitioners will refer to secondary care or to a GP with a special interest in this field.

In this chapter we will consider the following.
- Meniscal injuries and development of OA.
- Cruciate and collateral ligaments.
- The use of arthroscopy.
- Knee effusions.
- The use of arthrocentesis.
- Experimental procedures to preserve or restore articular cartilage.
- Surgical operations for severe disabling OA:
  1 arthroplasty (especially for knee and hip OA);
  2 osteotomy;
  3 unicompartmental knee replacement;
  4 arthrodesis.

Meniscal injuries and development of osteoarthritis

There is now plenty of evidence to show that removal of the medial or lateral meniscus increases the risk of developing OA. Recently, work by Stefan Lohmander's group in Lund, Sweden, has confirmed earlier studies [1]. Around 50% of patients develop an X-ray diagnosis of OA within

19 years following meniscectomy. Lateral meniscectomy shows a higher incidence of OA than for the medial meniscectomy. Interestingly, the contralateral knee also showed an increased incidence compared to controls.

Cruciate and collateral ligaments

The knee is a superbly engineered joint and a normal knee is able to absorb and deflect stresses throughout and around the joint. We know that damage to major knee structures leads to the development of OA in a high percentage of patients. If there is damage to, or rupture, of the cruciate ligaments, there is a far greater risk of OA developing because the smooth sliding, gliding motion of the knee is lost.

Severe injuries often involve all internal structures and even the collateral ligaments. We know that the quadriceps muscle protects the knee from sustaining damage, especially the vastus medialis part. If the bulk and quality of the muscle is good enough, this protection will make up for the loss of these knee components. There are some well-known footballers and rugby players maintaining a quality professional career in these situations. It is assumed that as their muscles become weaker, they may develop an accelerated form of OA, but only careful, prospective studies will answer this question.

The use of arthroscopy

Arthroscopy is both a diagnostic tool and a surgical treatment. Partial meniscectomies are performed through this scope, as are many anterior cruciate ligament repairs. The arthroscopist is in great demand, not just for these procedures but also for debridements and joint washouts.

The relief from pain following debridement and washout is extremely variable, being between 2 and 18 months. The shorter term relief raises the possibility of a strong placebo effect of the procedure. There are few adequately performed controlled trials of these arthroscopic procedures.

Arthroscopy is a surgical procedure with the usual list of possible scenarios. It is sensible to have a healthy scepticism of its role in patients with non-complicated OA.

Knee effusions

Knee effusions may occur following injury to the joint. We have already discussed 'Red Flags' (see pp. 19–21) and urgent advice for the most severe problems. It is important to aspirate any post-traumatic effusion to see whether blood is present. Joints do not like blood in their synovial fluid as it may cause adhesions and lead to flexion/extension deformities. Blood usually signifies more severe injuries and, invariably, a further opinion is necessary. In acute situations, removing this fluid will also relieve a lot of the pain.

Synovial effusions

A synovial effusion signifies that the joint has been damaged. The fluid is straw coloured. This may be from injuries or be caused by the OA itself. As a general principle, a synovial effusion signifies underlying cartilage damage. There may be a small to moderate recurrent effusion in a sportsperson, when there will be inevitable loss of quadriceps bulk. The effusion should alert us to suspect a meniscal injury. It is important to remember that this scenario may also occur in patients with OA. Very large effusions may be seen in patients with severely deranged knees. All these knees will have very poorly functioning quadriceps.

Arthrocentesis

When should a synovial effusion be drained?

To aid diagnosis

- To exclude an infected joint.
- To exclude a haemarthrosis (if there is blood in the joint it should be removed).
- To exclude or confirm crystal arthropathy.

To reduce pain and restriction of movement

- Knees with severe OA.
- Patients with comorbidities which exclude arthroplasty.
- These effusions are usually recurrent.
- Quantity of fluid removed varies from 50 to 150 ml.
- When excessive and recurrent consider referral for a medical synovectomy (i.e. using yttrium) or surgical synovectomy through an arthroscope.

*To treat flares of OA in those with moderate effusions
(less than 50 ml)*

- May be seen in patients who have a flare of their OA.
- May be no obvious cause.
- May follow increased unaccustomed activity.
- Joint may feel warm, but not hot.
- Infection may need to be excluded.
- Usually worthwhile instilling steroid and lidocaine, if there is no infection.
- There is evidence that simple arthrocentesis alone has a beneficial effect on pain and mobility [2].

Minimal effusions and dry osteoarthritic joints

If arthrocentesis is performed correctly on a knee joint, which has OA but no clinical effusion, in the great majority of joints it will be possible to remove a quantity of synovial fluid. This volume will vary from 0.5 to 15 ml. To obtain this fluid it will be necessary to push any fluid from behind and above the patella into the lateral and medial gutters of the knee. Next, squeeze the fluid from the opposite gutter into the gutter with the needle. The needle itself may become blocked and require rotation. Sometimes, even a small quantity of the fluid, already obtained, may need to be pushed back down the needle to unblock the needle bore. The bevelled needle, as it enters through the joint capsule, probably causes this blockage or valve effect.

Arthrocentesis and hyaluronans

Work from Nottingham University [3] has shown that only 60% of arthrocenteses of the knee joint are correctly placed. Correct placement of an arthrocentesis is probably more important today with the advent of the use of joint lubricants such as hyaluronans and the higher molecular weight derivatives, hylans. For these products to work they must be placed in the joint and not just close to the joint capsule. The Nottingham paper would be another explanation as to why the clinical studies of these products advocated a course of injections.

Accurate injections into abnormal joints, which are often misshapen and have loss of joint space, are not easy. Are injection techniques as accurate as we presume them to be? Perhaps fewer injections would be necessary, particularly with the hyaluronan preparations, if we could be sure that the injections could be correctly placed. This issue needs to

9

be addressed as the giving of fewer injections has practical and economic advantages.

Approaches to preserving and restoring articular cartilage

Arthroscopic debridement, ligament repair and use of hyaluronans or hylans are all undertaken to preserve or stimulate regeneration of articular cartilage. Often, they provide only temporary pain relief. They buy time and may give acceptable relief from severe pain. This may produce good pain management and allow continuous improvements in quality of life. Only well-conducted studies (including patient assessments) will help decide their place in the management of OA.

Experimental procedures

These are in an early stage of development and include grafting of bone, cartilage, periosteum and other constituents of the bone and cartilage joint interface. No evidence exists to show that they are of benefit in the OA knee.

Who should be referred to orthopaedic surgeons?

In simple terms, all patients who because of their arthritis:
- cannot sleep;
- cannot walk;
- cannot work.

This is discussed in Chapter 5. As primary care doctors we should be referring those patients who have severe pain, functional disability and structural joint damage for consideration of surgery, especially arthroplasty. The most important parameter is pain. Less weight should be given to disability and joint damage. Surgeons, historically, have relied upon X-ray changes, even though there may be large discrepancies between symptoms and X-ray changes.

The North of England survey [4] estimated that 2% of people aged 55 years or older might benefit from knee surgery. Interestingly, an American survey also concluded that knee replacement surgery was underutilized.

The North of England postal survey found that 8% of the population over 55 years old had knee pain and some disability. The 2% who had severe pain and disability, and might benefit from knee surgery, had seen

9

Patient name (last name, first name) .... Birth date (yy-mm-dd) ....
Patient address, phone ....
Date of referral .... Referring doctor .... Practice ....
....

Patient data

    Male ☐   Female ☐   Age .... Height (m) ....   Weight (kg) ....

Disease History

How long has this patient been symptomatic	Less than a year ☐	1–5 years ☐	Longer ☐
Major knee injury	Yes ☐	No ☐	Specify ....
Arthroscopy	Yes ☐	No ☐	Specify ....
Knee surgery	Yes ☐	No ☐	Specify ....

Current symptoms

Pain on walking	Yes ☐	No ☐
Pain at rest	Yes ☐	No ☐
Pain at night	Yes ☐	No ☐
Giving way	Yes ☐	No ☐
Grating	Yes ☐	No ☐
Swelling	Yes ☐	No ☐

Function

Occupation		
Condition affects employment	Yes ☐	No ☐
Able to walk indoors	Yes ☐	No ☐
Able to walk outdoors more than 1 km	Yes ☐	No ☐
Living alone	Yes ☐	No ☐
Carer for someone	Yes ☐	No ☐

Non-surgical treatments tried

Physiotherapy	Yes ☐	No ☐
Analgesics / non-steroidal anti-inflammatory drugs	Yes ☐	No ☐
Injections	Yes ☐	No ☐
Walking aids / insoles, etc.	Yes ☐	No ☐

Medical conditions that might influence surgery

	Yes ☐	No ☐
If yes, please specify		
Previous pulmonary embolism	Yes ☐	No ☐
Previous deep venous thrombosis	Yes ☐	No ☐

Other

Please provide a weight bearing X-ray (AP or PA view), taken within the last 12 months, with this form

I would like feedback and advice about the outcome of the consultation	Yes ☐	No ☐
Patient-completed WOMAC score sheet is attached with this form	Yes ☐	No ☐

9

Fig. 9.1 Knee OA referral form. This form is for use when referring patients for consideration for knee OA surgery.

their GP but few patients had been referred to secondary care, and fewer still were on a waiting list for surgery.

It would appear that attitudes of patients and doctors have a major influence on a patient's decisions to seek help or on a doctor's decision to refer (see Chapter 6). To improve both the appropriateness and quality of referral decisions, guidelines are being encouraged. Figure 9.1 is a model for the knee that could be used as a basis for local discussion. The referral is based around the everyday questions primary care doctors ask their patients and will allow an orthopaedic department to prioritize referrals. The referral also includes a patient-centred assessment (WOMAC, see Chapter 5 and Appendix 2) which has been validated and would be a valuable addition, especially if used in conjunction with the same assessment postoperatively. Obviously, similar forms may be compiled for hip OA.

Surgical operations

Arthroplasties

Arthroplasties transform lives and they are increasingly being performed. The number of arthroplasties performed varies greatly between different countries and communities. In the USA, hip arthroplasties may have peaked. It is unlikely that this has happened in the UK even though the current rate is well over 1 per 1000 of those aged over 65. In 1994–95 around 50 000 hip arthroplasties were performed. In the USA, rates for knee arthroplasties are now over 2 per 1000 of those aged over 65. In the UK they are well below this, being about half those of hip replacements, i.e. a rate between 0.5 and 0.7 per 1000 people aged over 65.

The pressure on orthopaedic surgeons to perform hip and knee operations is tremendous. It may be that the total number of hip operations will not rise much further but knee operation numbers have a very long way to go. It has been suggested that more knee operations will be required compared to hips. At present, the majority of patients have to wait a considerable time for their operation, leaving them with further reduced functional ability with the associated loss of mobility and independence. This may mean loss of abilities and hobbies so the patient becomes housebound or even chairbound. Postoperatively, few of these patients are likely to return to their more active roles and hobbies. Primary care doctors may compound these problems by being reluctant to refer patients, as waiting lists are long. Surgeons tend to defer obese patients though there is no research to show that the surgical outcomes are affected by obesity. However, anaesthetic risks and postoperative morbidity may be greater. Other patients may never be referred because of comorbidities. Patients taking non-steroidal anti-inflammatory drugs (NSAIDs) for their OA may be compounding these comorbidities. It is probable that with modern anaesthetics these decisions should be taken by a perioperative team and not by primary care or orthopaedic surgeons. To answer some of these questions we require large, pragmatic trials comparing surgical intervention with conservative therapy.

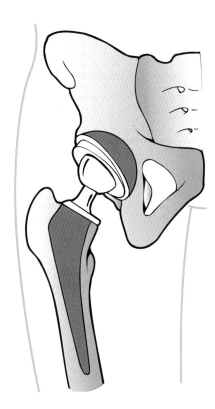

Fig. 9.2 Hip arthroplasty. From [6] with permission.

Hip arthroplasty

The Charnley type, low-friction arthroplasty (LFA) is the most commonly used cemented prosthesis (Fig. 9.2). It combines low wear and low friction by using metal on high-density polyethylene and using acrylic cement for both the acetabular cup and femoral shaft. This cement has to carry the shearing forces from the arthroplasty to the bone. These forces are high and ways of making and mixing the cement have been developed to increase its strength. Many other refinements have been made, but basically, Charnley got most things right—even down to the correct size of the femoral head.

Modern production techniques allow perfect matching ball-and-socket pairs, so that now there is a new interest in ceramic and metal on metal articulations. These have minimal wear compared to the metal on plastic implants (0.1–0.2 mm/year) and give the potential of longer implant life as well as low friction.

The only implants that have been thoroughly evaluated in the UK are the cheaper, standard, cemented implants such as the Charnley and the Stanmore [5]. These give the lowest, long-term failure rates (over

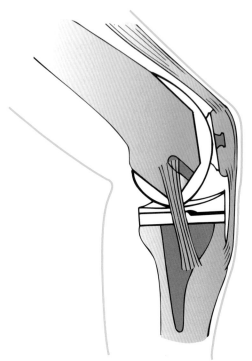

Fig. 9.3 Knee arthroplasty. From [6] with permission.

10–20 years). Other implants are too new for any medium/long-term assessments to have taken place.

Knee arthroplasty

A total knee prosthesis (tri-compartmental) is used in which the femoral component is anatomically shaped and uncemented fixation is used. The tibial component is modular. The metal base is fixed with cement and usually has a central peg or pegs helping stability. The polyethylene component fits into the tibial metal base. The patella may be resurfaced with a disc of polyethylene cemented to the resected joint surface of the patella. The surfaces of the prosthesis are incongruent, and most of its stability is provided by the ligaments and muscles (Fig. 9.3).

There are designs to try to decrease the high contact stresses and to increase congruent contact. All must include articulation for flexion, extension and axial rotation. The hope is to produce implants with low sheer force and low wear, so prolonging implant life.

Other arthroplasty operations

Hip and knee arthroplasties are the main operations performed for OA. We know that there are replacements for almost all peripheral joints; these having being developed for joints destroyed by inflammatory arthritis (e.g. rheumatoid arthritis). These operations are rarely indicated for patients with OA. Osteotomies and operations to possibly prevent or delay OA progression are discussed below.

Shoulder arthroplasty gives partial pain relief. Rarely is mobility returned as the rotator cuff and shoulder muscles are usually wasted.

The first metatarsophalangeal joint has had many experimental arthroplasties. None have been successful and the safe methods of arthrodesis and osteotomy remain the operations of choice.

We have already discussed hand OA and how rarely function loss is severe enough to warrant surgery (Chapter 5).

How long do replacement joints last?

Hip replacements have a 10-year 90% success rate, and 75% are functioning well after 15 years. Today's problem is the actual total number of operations, presently running at 50 000/year and rising. In comparison to hips, knee replacements have not been performed for so long, but do appear to have a similar life expectancy of between 10 and 15 years (Fig. 9.4). Interestingly, the 5-year survival rates of knee replacements are now better than for hips—a point that has been poorly communicated to the public and the medical profession. Sweden has recorded statistics for over 20 years. Figure 9.4 shows graphs of the improvements in survivals of total knee replacements.

Complications of hip and knee arthroplasty

Modern anaesthetics and early mobilization have greatly reduced the complications of surgery. The commonest complication is a deep vein thrombosis—even the incidence of these has been greatly reduced over the last few years. Other related complications have been reduced by perioperative antibiotic prophylaxis and improved surgical techniques.

The Swedish National Arthroplasty Register for Hips gives the accumulative revision rate of 0.6% for infection at 10 years. Haematogenous spread from other foci, e.g. urinary tract, gall bladder, lungs or dental abscess, is said to account for less than half this figure. Loosening is the major cause of revision, being about 10% at 10 years.

9

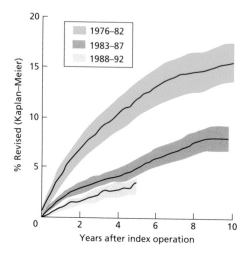

Fig. 9.4 Improvement of revision rates for total knee arthroplasty. From [6] with permission.

Complications of revision operations are higher and these operations take more time. There is an on-going debate as to whether revisions should be centralized to specialized clinics. This centralization may be encouraged with the development of large primary care cooperatives and other health-care reorganizations.

Osteotomy (Fig. 9.5)

The aim of an osteotomy is to reduce the loads on the most severely affected areas of the joint and transfer these stresses to areas with more articular cartilage. The operation also relieves pain and joint dysfunction and corrects malalignment. Both hip and knee joint osteotomies are undertaken. The principles are the same for both; the knee osteotomy will be considered here.

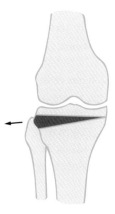

Fig. 9.5 Tibial (valgus) osteotomy: diagram showing bony wedge to be removed. From [6] with permission.

The lateral osteotomy is aimed at medial compartment knee OA. It must be done as a precision operation (similar to a joint replacement) and will redistribute the static and dynamic load on the articular surfaces. It gives excellent functional improvement as well as long-term pain relief. Importantly, it does not interfere with the patient's own knee joint so giving the option of a knee arthroplasty at a later date (Fig. 9.5).

The operation is quite demanding, mentally and physically, compared to a joint replacement. These demands include a longer hospital stay and longer rehabilitation. It is important to select the right patient (and the right surgeon). The results may give up to 10 years of pain relief, with maintenance of work, activities and hobbies.

Which patients to select for osteotomy

The best results are obtained by selecting patients who have severe knee pain and high activity demands, with early stage, or moderately advanced medial unicompartmental OA. For example, a farmer who wishes to continue farming (most farming involves high impact and high activity) or a person whose hobbies are very active, e.g. an enthusiastic skier or hill walker. The age of the patient is less of a barrier than activity and general fitness. The person should have an activity age of a 60-year-old or less.

Results of studies of beneficial effects of osteotomy

The percentages in Table 9.1 are the 'survival' rates of the operation. Poor pain relief or the return of severe pain (and disability) are the commonest reasons to convert the osteotomy to an arthroplasty.

Exclusion criteria for osteotomy

Certain factors will influence the success of the operation, mostly by exclusion.
- Loss of cruciate ligaments (loss of stability).
- Severe patellofemoral disease.
- Severe lower leg malalignment.

Table 9.1 Results of studies of the beneficial effects of osteotomy.

Hips		Knees	
1 year	90%	2 years	90%
5 years	70%	3–5 years	50–85%
10 years	30%	9 years+	15–57%

- Mentally or physically frail patients.
- 'Activity age' of over 60 years.
- Severe tibiofemoral disease.
- Advanced obesity.

Overall results for osteotomy vary much more than for joint replacement and even optimal candidates who initially have a good outcome tend, over time, to develop recurrent pain and loss of function. This can make it more difficult to advise the individual patient on which procedure to consider. Though, as stated above, an osteotomy does not preclude an arthroplasty at a later date.

Unicompartmental (unicondylar) knee replacement

Until recently this has had a very limited place, as few patients fit the recommended requirements, namely medial or lateral compartment disease with moderate or severe pain, and functional impairment. The remaining compartment should still be relatively intact. Importantly, there should be little patellofemoral disease or malalignment, and the cruciates should be intact. There is no upper age limit, but younger patients should be considered for an osteotomy.

Unicompartment implants have been less favoured by some surgeons, probably because the figures for loosening are about twice as high as for the total knee replacement and they do not appear to have improved. Unicompartmental knee replacements have a much higher revision rate: at 10 years it is well above 10%. Younger patients have a higher activity and a higher risk of loosening, but it should be remembered that revision of a failed unicompartmental implant is less complex than for a total knee replacement.

The procedure is being re-evaluated for the more elderly and frailer patients, as it is less demanding on them, both mentally and physically. The operation is quicker than for an arthroplasty; the hospital stay can be as short as a day. This means quicker mobilization and return to 'independence' and less likelihood of disorientation and other problems.

Arthrodesis

This operation 'fixes' the bones across a joint thus making the involved joint and bones a strong lever. In rheumatoid arthritis we see this quite often across wrist joints where the disease itself has ankylosed the bones and joints. An arthrodesis may be performed upon a failed knee or hip arthroplasty. Some patients request information about this operation, and the consequences of a completely failed or infected arthroplasty, before they will agree to the specific joint replacement. This operation is a relatively simple one which will give a pain-free result and the patient will usually be able to have a better quality of life after the operation, providing that the other joints can compensate for the loss of movement.

The carpometacarpal thumb joints sometimes require arthrodesis to give the patient a pain-free joint, with usually only a limited loss of dexterity. Few osteoarthritic patients fit into this category (see Chapter 5).

Postoperative management

Patient management is ongoing and patient education must start at the point and time of referral. Most patients require reassurance and advice on what to expect from the specialist and which operations may be considered.

Keeping patients informed is essential and helps in the overall outcome of operations. Patients undergoing hip arthroplasty are mobilized rapidly and are almost pain-free from day 1—some hospitals even discharge patients at this stage. In contrast, knee arthroplasty has a much longer rehabilitation period and the pain can be quite severe in the days following the operation. Patients may have fluctuating pain over the following weeks and months, but at 1 year the results are excellent. This difference in rehabilitation must be explained, otherwise this negative, initial comparison may lead to depression and, of course, a negative advertisement to friends and relatives. We must emphasize that the overall results are just as good for knees as for hips. Good preoperative management enables patients to avoid complications postoperatively, allowing them to exercise and mobilize with confidence and minimal pain. All these measures ensure our patients realize the benefits of surgery and reach their optimal functional ability postoperatively.

Postoperative referral form for primary care

To facilitate postoperative rehabilitation, consideration may be given to a locally designed referral form. A specimen is shown in Fig. 9.6. The aim is to improve the quality of follow-up and aftercare. The form considers most of the problems that primary care doctors sometimes have difficulty answering or dealing with when confronted by patient's questions or problems. It covers such things as physiotherapy, range of movements, walking aids and it answers questions, for example, about driving and about expected functional gain.

Coordination of discharges is extremely important in today's world of early mobilization and transfer to the community. Some essential

Patient name (last name, first name)................................. Birth date (yy-mm-dd) ....
Patient address, phone ....
Date of referral............................... Referring doctor...................... Practice ....

Patient data   Male ☐   Female ☐   Age ....

Operation   Date of operation .... Length of hospital stay .... days
    Arthroscopy   ☐
    Osteotomy   ☐
    Unicompartmental arthroplasty   ☐
    Bi/tricompartmental arthroplasty   ☐
    Other type of surgery   ☐   Specify...............................
    Post-operative complications   infection ☐ deep vein thrombosis ☐   PE ☐
                                    other   ☐   Specify...............................

Rehabilitation and follow-up suggested
    Specific rehabilitation   Yes ☐   No ☐   Time.......... weeks
    Physiotherapy   Yes ☐   No ☐   Time.......... weeks
    Use of walking aid   Yes ☐   No ☐   Time.......... weeks
    Wound treatment   Yes ☐   No ☐   Specify................. Time ...... weeks
    Calf/knee swelling treatment Yes ☐   No ☐   Specify................. Time ...... weeks
    Anti-thrombotic therapy   Yes ☐   No ☐   Specify................. Time ...... weeks

Patient activity and expected outcome of surgery
    Expected range of movement   .... degrees
    Possible minor complications   pain ☐ for............weeks   swelling ☐ for........ weeks
    Full weight bearing expected   now ☐ after......... weeks
    Patient may drive car   now ☐ after......... weeks
    Expected functional gain at 6 months ....

    Patient must NOT do impact sports or heavy work

General information
    Patient must be reminded that after arthroplasty the knee is expected to be stable and pain free, but that the knee will not be a normal knee

Fig. 9.6 Knee OA, postoperative referral form. This form is for referring a patient who has recently undergone knee OA surgery back to primary care. The function of this form is to improve the quality of follow-up and aftercare.

areas of this care are discussed below, mainly to help to prevent problems arising and to improve rehabilitation services.

Points to remember

• Good analgesia postoperatively will facilitate rapid postoperative mobilization.

• Patients may need a prescription or advice on their drug regime especially concerning pain relief.

• Active exercises (as well as passive movements) will begin as soon as possible. These will increase strength, voluntary control and re-establish normal gait and balance.

- Before patients are discharged from hospital they should be safe on stairs. Movements should be free. For knees there should be full, active extension and at least 90° of flexion. Hospital physiotherapists usually deal with this.
- Written instructions should be given to patients and their carers so that the patient can be encouraged to continue simple exercises at home. It is essential for them to understand what to do and how often.

Points for the patient and carers to remember

- The patient's exercise regime should be fully understood.
- The patient's ability to perform these exercises should be understood.
- What goals the patient should have should be listed and understood.
- During recovery at home patients should be given adequate social support. They need advice on what to do and when to seek help. Many hospitals have an advice helpline for the use of both patients and doctors.
- Some understanding of the anticipated time scale of progression is necessary. For instance, it is important to realize that improvement can continue for up to 1–2 years. This is especially so for knee replacements.
- If the joint becomes painful and swollen, apply ice and temporarily decrease the exercise regime. It needs to be pointed out that prolonged immobilization increases the risk of postoperative complications, especially muscle atrophy, leading to a decreased range of movements which may impede overall attainment.
- Any potential problems and pitfalls should be listed and understood.

Summary points

- Meniscal problems can appear in arthritic joints.
- Meniscectomy may lead to OA on X-ray in 50% of patients.
- Arthroscopy may only have short-term benefits.
- Arthrocentesis is often beneficial.
- Hip and knee arthroplasties transform lives.
- Long-term survival of implants continues to increase.
- Infection rates are less than 1%.
- Loosening is 10% or less at 10 years for both hip and knee arthroplasties.
- Knees have a longer rehabilitation time than hips.
- Knee results are now as good as hip arthroplasties.

References

1   Roos H, Lauren M, Roos E, Adalberth T, Lohmander S. Risk factors and osteoarthrosis after meniscectomy. *Arthritis Rheum* 1998 41 (Suppl. 9), abstract 326.

2   Miller JH, White J, Norton TH. The value of intra-articular injections in osteoarthritis of the knee. *J Bone Joint Surg* 1958; 40B: 363–643.

3   Jones A, Regan M, Ledingham J, Pattrick M., Manhire A, Doherty M. Importance of placement of intra-articular steroid injections. *BMJ* 1993; 307: 1329–30.

4   Tennant A, Fear J, Pickering A *et al*. Prevalence of knee problems in the population aged 55 years and over: identifying the need for knee arthroplasty. *BMJ* 1995; 310: 1291–3.

5   Total hip replacement. *Bulletin: Effective Health Care* 1996; Volume 2 No. 7.

6   Brandt KD, Doherty M, & Lohmander LS. *Osteoarthritis*. Oxford: Oxford University Press, 1998.

9

CHAPTER 10

Long-term Management and Referral

There are huge numbers of patients with osteoarthritis (OA). These numbers are increasing as the population ages. Many of these patients have learned to live with their joint pain and have adapted their lives accordingly. The vast majority do not come to see their primary care doctor on a regular basis but cope by simple adaptations and by taking over-the-counter analgesics. Sometimes these patients will come for reassurance about the diagnosis, and once their GP has seen and advised on this, they are happy to continue to cope on their own. Patients often put up with increasing loss of function without seeking medical help, but increasing pain usually prompts patients to attend their GP. They then present for reassurance, help with pain control or general advice. At this stage it may still be appropriate to manage these patients within primary care, with appropriate advice, reassurance and simple drug therapy, as previously discussed.

Pain management strategies

For many years it was known that inflammatory joint disease gave symptoms of severe pain whereas the pain of OA was thought to be much less demanding. A survey of 500 OA patients undertaken by the authors in two general practices, one urban and one rural, showed that pain relief was the single biggest problem that these patients had. The results showed that 80% of patients coped with everyday activities with no difficulty or some difficulty. These simple tasks included dressing and undressing, getting in and out of bed, walking on the flat and climbing five steps. However, 40% of patients with OA experienced some difficulty in sleeping because of pain and over 30% were unable to control the pain of their OA. Many patients felt that their doctors underestimated the pain of their OA.

Pain is subjective and none of us know what someone else is experiencing in terms of pain. It is often tempting to respond to a patient's distress by continually increasing or changing the analgesia for those who come back time after time saying that nothing is helping. When this is the case, instead of repeatedly changing treatment, it is important to review the whole clinical picture.

Reassessment options

- Reassess the clinical history and the patient's specific symptoms and comorbidities.
- Perform a full examination of the affected joint(s).
- Check whether there are any other social or psychological factors operating.
- Assess whether the patient is depressed.
- Consider using a simple cognitive or behavioural approach to pain control.
- Consider whether some different treatment strategy would be helpful, such as physiotherapy, an intra-articular injection and possibly referral to a pain clinic for acupuncture or a transcutaneous electrical nerve stimulation (TENS) machine.

Patients with stable, chronic disease often become regular attenders at the primary care doctor and may ask for different treatments on a repeating basis. Often, having taken a full history, the doctor may find that the patient has not complied with the previous treatment but is, nevertheless, demanding something further. This kind of behaviour may reflect poor communication between doctor and patient, poor education of the patient by the doctor or primary care team or the patient's distress at coping with chronic, painful and debilitating disease.

It may be that there is a clinical problem—perhaps the joint has deteriorated to such an extent that surgery may need to be considered. The pain of hip or knee OA in a badly damaged joint can be very severe and should not be underestimated. If such patients are awaiting surgery and standard analgesics and non-steroidal anti-inflammatory drugs are not effective, perhaps we should consider small doses of opiates as pain relief prior to surgery. Such patients in severe pain find that joint replacement surgery provides huge relief from pain and the patients can then manage without strong pain killers and their associated problems of addiction.

Pain cannot be treated as an isolated factor. Patients with severe OA require considerable social support and this may be through the primary care team, hospital outpatients, social services or one of the patient support groups.

Referral within the community

Some patients may require referral, not necessarily to secondary care but to one of a number of other options. The outcome of such a referral may be sufficient to provide ongoing support for the patient (Fig. 10.1).

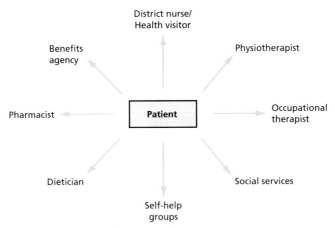

Fig. 10.1 Referral options within the community.

Referral to secondary care

At times patients may need to be referred to secondary care for a number of reasons.
- To confirm diagnosis.
- To help with management.
- Because of patient pressure.

Diagnostic reasons

The majority of patients with OA will be relatively easy to diagnose in primary care but there will be instances when the diagnosis is not clear. The outcome of such a referral may be a single visit to confirm the diagnosis and suggest a management plan or regular outpatient attendance for ongoing assessment and treatment.

Management reasons

Management reasons for referral to secondary care include the following.
- Access to resources: some specialist resources may not be available within the community and the patients may need to be referred to access these services, e.g. investigation, physiotherapy, occupational therapy, acupuncture, aids and appliances.
- Patients may be referred for a specialist technique, e.g. some form of injection therapy, which the primary care doctor may not feel confident in using.

• Consideration for surgery: patients with OA may be referred to an orthopaedic surgeon for consideration for a surgical procedure, such as a joint washout, an osteotomy or a total joint replacement.

• Increasing pain: in these circumstances patients may be referred to a rheumatologist or to a specialized pain clinic for drug therapy, injection therapy or to a pain psychologist or to take part in a pain management programme, with cognitive and behavioural approaches.

Patient pressure

In some instances this is a valid reason for referral, even though the primary care doctor does not feel that anything can be achieved by this referral. Patients with chronic, painful conditions, such as OA, sometimes lose faith in their primary care doctor and feel that they need to see a specialist. This can often be helpful, as it will usually back up the management of the primary care doctor and reassure the patient that all that should be done is being done. Alternatively, secondary care may have something else to offer in terms of specialist physiotherapy or pain relief.

Alternative or complementary therapy

No matter how supportive and well informed the doctor might be, patients with chronic disease, such as OA, often look for help outside the treatments of conventional medicine, as they may have found little benefit from standard management. These patients often ask whether complementary medicine would help their OA. It is sometimes difficult to answer this. There is very little scientific evidence proving a benefit for most of these treatments but there is no doubt that some patients find benefit from receiving treatments such as homeopathy, acupuncture, herbal medicine, chiropractic techniques, osteopathy, aromatherapy and so on. There may be several reasons for this apparent benefit.

• The complementary practitioner can often give more time to the patient.

• The service costs money and this is often psychologically important (if you pay for it, it must be good).

• There is a 'mystique' to the treatment, which many patients may find appealing.

• The treatment is free of 'nasty drugs'.

• The treatment may work!

The provision of complementary or alternative medicine varies greatly from area to area and it is said that there are more complementary therapists than GPs in the UK. Some areas have units dealing in complementary medicine attached to NHS hospitals and alternative therapies are now available in an increasing number of GP surgeries.

A recent survey showed that more than a quarter of patients attending rheumatology and orthopaedic outpatient departments, had already tried complementary therapies and half of these patients said that they had gained some benefit.

There is now some statutory regulation of some branches of complementary medicine, following the establishment of the General Osteopathic Council and the General Chiropractic Council. Although there is, as yet, only inconclusive evidence of both effectiveness and cost-effectiveness, there are increasing numbers of studies looking at the way these therapies may work.

Where conventional medicine might use pharmacological therapies, alternative medicine may use nutritional therapies, homeopathy or herbal medicine. Where conventional medicine may use biomechanical approaches, such as physiotherapy and surgery, alternative medicine may use osteopathy, chiropractic techniques and acupuncture. Where conventional medicine may use clinical psychology and patient education, alternative medicine may use hypnotherapy and various other sensory therapies, although in any one patient, there would probably be a mixture of therapies to give a holistic approach, both in conventional and alternative therapies.

There are a number of negative aspects to alternative and complementary therapy. Practitioners of these therapies may have variable professional training and they do not have to swear the Hippocratic Oath. Conventional practitioners rarely receive any feedback from alternative therapists. It can be disconcerting for a patient to tell you that they have recently had an X-ray, for example of the lower back, from an alternative therapist, without any reference in the patient's NHS file. I neither encourage nor discourage my patients from trying such treatments. Most alternative therapies rarely do harm and many may do some short-term good, if only to decrease tension and make the patient more relaxed, and perhaps more confident about their condition. When the patient ceases to feel benefit, he or she will discontinue the treatment of their own accord. Although many patients try such treatments in the short term, very few continue to attend on a long-term basis.

Self-help groups

Although doctors do not officially refer patients to self-help groups, it is certainly worth telling patients about these groups and encouraging them to self-refer and to find out more about the innovative arthritis self-management programmes being set up.

Chronic care

The management of patients with chronic, painful illness is a major challenge for primary care doctors. These conditions are not life-threatening and do not respond to dramatic interventions and doctors may become dispirited at the thought of regular consultations with patients for whom they seem to be doing very little. Looking after these patients, and maintaining confidence and a positive attitude, is undoubtedly a difficult task but doing this well is a sign of a caring and compassionate doctor.

10

CHAPTER 11

Economic and Research Considerations

We have continued to emphasize that osteoarthritis (OA) is not caused by age but is associated with ageing. Ageing puts a higher proportion of the population at risk of OA. This is important when we consider OA from an economic point of view, in relation to the country's gross national product (GNP) and the impact it has on the national economy and society in general.

The costs of OA appear to be equally shared between direct expenditure for medical care services and the indirect impact of OA on society. This probably applies to most countries with Western-type economies and will probably remain so. Unfortunately, there is a lack of concern about OA leading to a lack of evidence-based studies. OA is costly as it has a high prevalence, with a high to moderate impact on society and the medical services. Costs of OA outstrip rheumatoid arthritis (RA) costs by at least 50%. In the USA the on-going cost of arthritis is equivalent to a moderate recession (2.5% of GNP) year on year; the difference being that recessions do not last for ever.

The American Federal Government annual community-based surveys give the figure of 12.3% for the prevalence of OA in the community. This compares with 6% prevalence based on a doctor's examination.

Doctor assessments will always underestimate the size of the problem, as it is probable that at least 40% of people with OA, of a similar severity to the diagnosed population, do not present to a doctor. This is borne out by community surveys on back pain, as well as musculoskeletal conditions, in the UK (see Table 11.1).

Table 11.1 Who treats: GP or self?			
Complaint	Visit GP (millions)	Self-treat (millions)	Total (millions)
Muscle aches	1.2 (12%)	8.8 (88%)	10.0 (100%)
Back problems	1.4 (25%)	4.2 (75%)	5.6 (100%)
Sprains/strains	1.4 (34%)	2.7 (66%)	4.1 (100%)

How do we look at the costs of osteoarthritis?

We should consider the costs from two major viewpoints.
- Direct expenditure for medical care services:
    1 secondary care;
    2 primary care;
    3 complementary medicine.
- Indirect impact of illness on an individual's function in society:
    1 loss of wages;
    2 loss of caring and the helper role (becoming dependent rather than independent);
    3 need for carers/caring;
    4 loss of leisure and hobbies and related activities due to the disease or its associates (e.g. depression, isolation).

These latter activities are difficult to evaluate financially but have a major effect on an individual's quality of life and well-being.

Reducing costs

The reduction of costs can be considered from three main areas.
- Reducing hospital costs—especially reducing hospital admissions for surgical procedures.
- Looking at the impact of OA on the workplace—loss of wages, on carers and caring.
- Other direct medical costs—especially drugs and visits to doctors and complementary practitioners.

It is important to relate costs on an individual patient basis, as we can equate these figures more easily. Total global figures are so astronomically large that they become almost meaningless. This does not help to individualize costs, or create the right environment for efficiencies in state-run systems.

Secondary care costs and evaluation

Studies are required to evaluate surgical procedures, not only against other procedures but also against medical management (both pharmacological and physical therapies). We need to emulate Sweden and instigate a national register for evaluating different prostheses and surgical performance. Only then will we be able to define centres and units of excellence, so possibly moving towards certification of centres (or individuals) for revision procedures. In this way, orthopaedic procedures and units will be able to produce statistics similar to perinatal and maternity ones.

11

Table 11.2 QALY costs as assessed by patients and surgeons for hip and knee arthroplasty.	Patient	Surgeon
Knee	£1399	£703
Hip	£500	£333

Cost and quality of life

Unfortunately, most medical interventions and surgical procedures need to be financially justified, as 'all' are competing for a finite amount of money.

Cost-effectiveness analysis for arthroplasty

Cost-effectiveness analysis in the UK and USA have shown these procedures to be highly cost-effective, as they do transform lives, giving a huge improvement in quality of life. Trying to put a cost to this involves using a measure called quality adjusted life years (QALY). Recent studies suggest that these operations compare favourably with other major procedures, such as coronary artery bypass grafting. Not surprisingly, this measure gives different costs when using patient or consultant evaluations. Orthopaedic surgeons are much more optimistic (Table 11.2).

The costs depend crucially on the length of survival of the implant. A 15-year survival transforms these estimates as costs (QALYs) for repeat operations are much higher than for the original operation.

Patient-centred outcomes

As previously mentioned, patient assessments are different and patient-based QALYs are more costly than those based on consultant assessment. Most outcome studies have been based around implant survival and few have contained patient-centred measures of outcome. Ninety per cent of patients report good or excellent outcomes after arthroplasty. This is a turn round from the 95% who had severe or moderate pain before operation. It is important to realize that patients may still experience pain following these operations. For instance, one in five patients experience moderate pain 7 years after knee arthroplasty.

Primary care problems

Patients derive pleasure from choice (and presumably improved outcome). It would seem that patients should be allowed some voice as to the level of individual health care they receive. This is because as

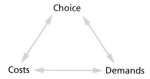

Fig. 11.1 As economies expand, the pressure for choice grows.

economies expand, the pressure for choice also grows (Fig. 11.1).

In the UK choice is more difficult as, in reality, the NHS is a nationalized industry and choice is controlled by finite costs. The Patient Charter and raising of patient expectations has not been a practical alternative. In fact, it has led to increased demands on primary care and primary care practitioners. It is not always possible to meet these expectations. Added to this has been a rising perception of a lack of benefit from conventional therapies and there has been an enormous rise in complementary practitioners. This has led to pressure for these practitioners to have a register both to facilitate patient access to them and set nationally recognizable standards.

The triangle of choice outlined in Fig. 11.1 between demands and costs is constantly changing. Different economies develop different answers, which also change with time.

Economic aspects of medical and non-medical approaches

We know that non-steroidal anti-inflammatory drugs (NSAIDs) decrease(s) symptoms of OA but we need critically to appraise the treatments used in OA. There is no evidence that they retard OA progress or prolong life though we have learnt the cost of their side-effects, both to the individual and to society (see Chapter 8). This means we are unable to undertake straightforward cost-effective analysis which looks at which therapy, for instance, prevented joint replacement or 'the years of life' extended by therapy.

Unfortunately, few studies are large enough to compare NSAIDs and analgesics and their effect on pain and function. We require large population studies, which look at these issues, as well as biomechanical and non-biomedicinal approaches. Hurley and Scott [1] showed that moderate physiotherapy has a beneficial effect on proprioception and quadriceps strength improving patient's well-being by decreasing their disability. This is an important study for primary care prevention of disability, especially when added to work from epidemiologists showing that the prediction of independence at age 76 (and beyond) is related to walking speed and muscle strength at age 70.

There is a need to conduct more studies on the economic impact of OA, so that we can plan adequately for the pandemic of OA that we face with the ageing population. As well as looking at the issues already mentioned, these studies should also consider the underutilization of surgical procedures, especially knee arthroplasty, and the impact of educational programmes on self-management.

Areas that warrant review and research

Medical research questions

- What is the safety of simple and compound analgesics?
- How does taking medication on an 'as required' basis affect costs and side-effects?
- What is the relative effectiveness and efficiency of topical NSAIDs and oral NSAIDs in patients with OA?
- Well-designed, large-scale, randomized trials comparing alternative therapies are required to evaluate physical, medical and complementary therapies. What effect do these treatments have on both pain and function?
- What is the role of COX 2 selective NSAIDs, nitrosated compounds and *Helicobacter pylori* infection in primary care treatment of patients with OA?

Surgical research issues

- Improving preoperative assessment and physical conditioning before operations.
- Possibilities for earlier discharge and continuing self-help and conditioning begun preoperatively.
- National registers for recording success rates etc. for different prostheses and surgeons. Sweden has an excellent system.
- Studies to define centres and units of excellence, thus helping considerations for certification of centres for revision procedures. In this way orthopaedic procedures and units will develop statistics similar to perinatal and maternity statistics.
- Ways of allowing patient choice and even financial contributions in medical and surgical treatments.

All of these issues rely on cooperation, education and, not least, the enthusiasm of primary care doctors. It will require primary care-based academic units with specific interest in musculoskeletal diseases. A good example is the unit developing around Keele.

11

Indirect impact of osteoarthritis

Some research has been undertaken to try to quantify some of the work-related problems of OA.
- 11% of people diagnosed with OA have reduced hours of work.
- 9% are unemployed.
- 14% retire early due to OA.

These figures are taken from a community survey of residents with a diagnosis of OA in Ormstead County, Minnesota [2]. It will naturally underestimate the impact, as it is probable that at least 40% of people with OA, of similar severity to the diagnosed population, do not present to a doctor. Similar percentages for common musculoskeletal problems are shown in Table 11.1.

Summary points

- OA costs to society and medical services are 50% greater than RA costs.
- OA costs are shared equally between direct expenditure on medical services and indirect costs on society.
- In expanding economies individuals expect more choice.
- More research is required into comparing medical and surgical treatments.

References

1 Hurley MV, Scott DL. Improvements in quadriceps sensorimotor function and disability of patients with knee osteoarthritis following a clinically practicable exercise regime. *Br J Rheumatol* 1998; 37: 1181–7.
2 Gabriel SE, Crowson CS, O'Fallon WM. Costs of osteoarthritis: estimates from a geographically defined population. *J Rheumatol Suppl* 1995; 43: 23–5.

'GALS' Screening Examination

This is a useful screening test to identify patients who may require a more detailed examination.

Initially ask three questions:
- Have you any pain or stiffness in your muscles, joints or back?
- Do you have trouble getting up or down stairs?
- Do you have difficulty getting dressed?

If the patient answers yes to any questions, proceed with a more detailed examination.

Gait Examine the patient walking away, turning and walking back.

Arms Inspect dorsum of hands, observe supination and inspect palmar aspect of hands, then check power grip and pinch grip; check full extension of elbow; ask the patient to put his/her hands behind the head; and up behind back as far as possible, apply the metacarpophalangeal squeeze test, and supraspinatus skinfold rolling test.

Legs Internal rotation of the hip with knee–hip flexion, inspection of the knee for swelling or quadriceps wasting; feel knee during flexion for crepitus, inspect soles of feet; metatarsophalangeal squeeze test.

Spine Examine from behind for scoliosis and leg length inequality, examine from the side for kyphosis and lordosis and ask the patient to touch his/her toes; examine from in front and ask the patient to put his/her ear on each shoulder.

For more in-depth GALS screening read—
- ARC Report from collected reports on Rheumatic Diseases 1995.

Reference

Doherty M, Dacre J, Dieppe P, Smith M. The GALS locomotor screen. *Rheum Dis* 1992; 51: 1165–9.

WOMAC (Western Ontario and MacMaster Universities Osteoarthritis Index) and Lequesne Scales

WOMAC [1]

This is a three-dimensional, self-administered measure specific to osteoarthritis (OA), looking at pain, stiffness and physical function in OA of hip or knee. The assessment formats are either a visual analogue scale or a Likert scale.

Visual analogue scale

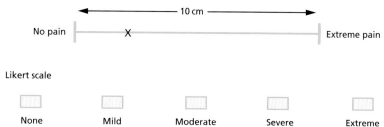

There are 24 questions, 5 on pain, 2 on stiffness and 17 on physical function.

Lequesne—algo-functional indices [2]

These are two indices, one for hip and one for knee, looking at pain, maximum distance walked and activities of daily living. These indices are more difficult for patients to self-administer than the WOMAC and may require an interviewer. Questions are asked and points allocated according to the patient's reply and a high score indicates greater severity, e.g.
- pain or discomfort during nocturnal bed rest:
  1 none or insignificant—0;
  2 only on movement or in certain positions—1;
  3 with no movement—2.

References

1 Bellamy N, Buchanan WW, Goldsmith CH *et al*. Validation Study of WOMAC: A health status instrument for measuring clinically important patient relevant outcomes to antirheumatic drug therapy in patients with osteoarthritis of the hip or knee. *J Rheumatol* 1998; 15: 1833–40.
2 Lequesne MG, Mery C, Samson M *et al*. Indexes of severity for osteoarthritis of the hip and knee: validation-value in comparison with other assessment tests. *Scand J Rheumatol* 1987; (Suppl. 65): 85–9.

2

Beighton Score

Classic signs of hypermobility

	Right	Left
Dorsiflexion of the 5th MCP to 90°	1	1
Apposition of thumb to volar aspect of forearm	1	1
Hyperextension of the elbow by 10°	1	1
Hyperextension of the knee by 10°	1	1
Hands flat on the floor with knees extended	1	
Total		**9 points**

Useful Addresses

Arthritis Care
18 Stephenson Way
London NW1 2HD, UK
Tel: 0171 916 1500
Fax: 0171 916 1505

Arthritis Research Campaign
Copeman House
St Mary's Gate
Chesterfield S41 7TD, UK
Tel: 01246 558033
Fax: 01246 558007

European League against Arthritis (EULAR)
Fred Wyss, Executive Secretary
Witikonerstrasse 15
Zurich
Switzerland
Tel: 0041 1383 9690
Fax: 0041 1383 9810

Primary Care Rheumatology Society
PO Box 42
Northallerton
North Yorkshire DL7 8YG, UK
Tel: 01609 774 794
Fax: 01609 774 726

The British Society for Rheumatology
41 Eagle Street
London WC1R 4AR, UK
Tel: 0171 242 3313
Fax: 0171 242 3277
http://www.rheumatology.org.uk

The American College of Rheumatology
1800 Century Place
Suite 250
Atlanta
Georgia 30345, USA
Tel: 001 404 633 377
Fax: 001 404 633 1870

University of Bath and PCR Diploma
University of Bath
Bath BA2 7AY, UK
Tel: 01225 826 878
Fax: 01225 826 849

4

Further Reading

Journal articles and other references

Barlow JH, Turner AP, Wright CC. Long-term outcomes of an arthritis self-management programme. *Br J Rheumatol* 1998; 37: 1315–19.
(An excellent study, from an initiative by Arthritis Care, showing the benefits of patient and community led self-management.)

Lorig KR, Mazonson PD, Holman HR. Evidence suggesting that health education for self-management in patients with chronic arthritis has sustained health benefits while reducing healthcare costs. *Arthritis Rheum* 1993; 36: (No. 4 April).
(The American experience of the good effect of self-management programmes on chronic arthritis. This is the classic paper from which self-management studies have evolved.)

Oxford Pain Research
http://www.ebando.com
(We have included a few references on OA management guidelines as most are soon out dated. We suggest that you regularly visit this free website which is kept up to date. It is evidence based from the internationally renowned Oxford Group who also run the evidence-based journal *Bandolier*.)

Moore AR, Phillips CJ. Cost of NSAID adverse effects to the UK National Health Service. *J Med Econ* 1999; 2: 45–55.
(An excellent review of the proper costs of NSAIDs adverse effects. This allows doctors to make rational decisions for individual patients using today's drugs and possibly extrapolate for newer ones.)

Dieppe P, Basler HD, Chard, J, *et al*. Knee replacement surgery for osteoarthritis: effectiveness, practice variations, indications and possible determinants of utilization. *Rheum* 1999; 38; 73–83.
(An excellent in-depth report which will make doctors review the whole of their OA practice not just knee problems.)

Felson DT, Zhang Y. An update on the epidemiology of knee and hip osteoarthritis with a view to prevention. *Arthritis Rheum* 1998; 41(8): 1343–55.

5

(A superb update from Felson of Framingham Study fame. A must if you want to be up to speed on factors which have a bearing on OA from genetics to tertiary prevention.)

Cushnaghan J, McCarthy C, Dieppe P. Tapping the patella medially: a new treatment for osteoarthritis of the knee joint? *BMJ* 1994; 308: 753–5. (Our grandmothers swaddled their knees—was it to change the patella tracking and relieve anterior pain? This is a simple treatment that may be tried.)

Hurley MV, Scott DL. Improvements in quadriceps sensorimotor function and disability of patients with knee osteoarthritis following a clinically practicable exercise regime. *Br J Rheum* 1998; 37: 1181–7.
(We know that quadriceps protect the knee, but we are unsure that research physiotherapy can be applied to everyday practice. This trial addresses the issue.)

Eccles M, Freemantle N, Mason J, *et al.* North of England evidence-based guideline development project: summary guideline for non-steroidal anti-inflammatory drugs versus basic analgesia in treating the pain of degenerative arthritis. The North of England Non-Steroidal Anti-Inflammatory Drug Guideline Development Group. *BMJ* 1998; 317: 526–36.
(The correct way to put evidence-based guidelines together using working GPs, academic experts and health economists from York.)

Guidelines for the diagnosis, investigation and management of osteoarthritis of the hip and knee. Report of a joint working group of the British Society of Rheumatology and the Research Unit of the Royal College of Physicians. *J R Coll Physicians Lond* 1993; 27(4).
(A good report but not many primary care doctors involved!)

Hochberg MC, Altman RD, Brandt KD *et al.* Guidelines for the Medical Management of Osteoarthritis. Part 1, Osteoarthritis of the hip. Part II Osteoarthritis of the knee. *Arthritis Rheum* 1995; 38(11): 1541–6.
(The original classic work of the ACR under Marc Hochberg. Worthwhile reading, even today.)

Bellamy N, Buchanan WW, Goldsmith CH *et al.* Validation study of WOMAC: a health status instrument for measuring clinically important patient relevant outcomes to antirheumatic drug therapy in patients with osteoarthritis of the hip or knee. *J Rheumatol* 1988; 15: 1833–40.
(Professor Nicolas Bellamy is the acknowledged world expert on instruments for OA measurements. Well validated and easy to use by patients and doctors to assess pain and disability.)

Lequesne MG, Mery C, Samson M *et al.* Indexes of severity for osteo-arthritis of the hip and knee: validation–value in comparison to other assessment tests. *Scand J Rheumatol* 1987 Suppl. 65; 85–9.
(Lequesne-initiated OA assessments. This supplement is easy to read and worthwhile.)

Books

Klippel JH, Dieppe PA. *Rheumatology*. London: Mosby-Yearbook (Europe) Ltd, 1999.
(Two large volumes, well illustrated and a phenomenal reference. Most good libraries keep a current volume.)

Silver T. *Joint and Soft Tissue Injections*, 2nd edn. Abingdon: Radcliffe Medical Press, 1999.
(An excellent short book from a primary care perspective. A worthwhile addition to a personal library.)

Snaith M. *ABC of Rheumatology*. London: BMJ Publishing Group, 1996.
(A quick, short reference book from the BMJ series of ABC. Covers most subjects with good pictures and diagrams.)

Dieppe P, Kirwan J, Cooper C, McGill N. *Arthritis and Rheumatism in Practice*, London: Gower Medical, 1990.
(Excellent short, well illustrated, practical approach to general practice rheumatology.)

Brandt KD, Doherty M, Lohmander LS. *Osteoarthritis*. Oxford: Oxford University Press, 1998.
(A good, very academic view of osteoarthritis.)

Klippel J, Dieppe P, Ferri FF. *Primary Care Rheumatology*. London: Mosby, 1999.
(A comprehensive, academic review with excellent illustrations and diagrams, well laid out.)

Diploma of Primary Care Rheumatology by Distance Learning. University of Bath and Primary Care Rheumatology Society.
(A very practical, general practice-based course for those taking a particular interest in primary care rheumatology. Written by GPs with advice being given by specialists.)

Useful Websites

Bandolier (provides links to many other useful websites).
http://www.ebando.com

Oxford Pain Research (includes listing of systematic reviews in pain relief).
http://www.ebando.com

Cochrane Collaboration.
http://hiru.mcmaster.ca/cochrane

University of York, NHS Centre for Reviews & Dissemination.
http://www.york.ac.uk/inst/crd/welcome.htm

Evidence Based Healthcare Resources (again good links to other useful sites).
http://www.northglashealthinfo.org.uk

Especially for searching

PubMed (database which includes citations not yet on MEDLINE).
http://www.ncbi.nlm.nih.gov/PubMed

WebSPIRS (internet access to ERL databases including MEDLINE, EMBASE etc.).
N.B. 30 days free trial but after that it costs to subscribe.
http://forge.silverplatter.com/webspirs/webspirs.htm

Dr Felix (links to all the free MEDLINE access around the world).
http://www.docnet.org.uk/drfelix/

Biomednet (databases including 'evaluated' MEDLINE).
N.B. free.
http://www.biomednet.com/gateways/db/medicine

BIDS (UK non-profitmaking database providers—home of EMBASE).
http://www.bids.ac.uk/

CISCOM (centralised information service for complementary medicine).
http://www.gn.apc.org/rccm/ciscom.htm

OMNI (Organising Medical Networked Information, provides search engine for various websites and access to MEDLINE).
http://omni.ac.uk/

iHEA (the International Health Economics Association is one of the world's premier health economics societies. Its page provides links to many of the websites involved in evidence based medicine).
http://www.healtheconomics.org/links/dissemination.htm

PCR (the Primary Care Rheumatology Society is a leading authority in primary care education in musculo-skeletal medicine).
http://www.pcrsociety.com

6

Index

Note: page numbers in *italics* refer to figures, those in **bold** refer to tables

abductor muscles 34, 36
acetaminophen 66
acromegaly 9
acromioclavicular joint 34, 38, 48, *49*, *50*
    painful arc *49*
Acupan 89
acupuncture 117, 119
adaptive aids 81
aetiology of OA 1
age, OA risk 9
ageing 121
aids
    and appliances 117
    environmental 82
    patient 81–3, *84*
allopurinol 27
alternative therapies 118–19, 122
American College of Rheumatology (ACR)
    definition of OA 56
    diagnostic guidelines 52, **53**
amitryptilene 89
analgesia
    postoperative 112
    TENS 80
analgesics 2
    compound **85**, 87–8
    pain management 66
    side-effects 88
    stronger 88–9
anserine bursa 36, *37*
    see also bursitis, anserine
antalgic gait 34, 36, 45
anterior knee pain 25, 39
anticoagulants 92
antidepressants **85**, 89
antiogensin-converting enzyme (ACE)
        inhibitors 92
apatite crystals, severe OA 5, 6, 100
apophyseal joints 52
arthralgia, viral 24
arthritis, septic 9, 10, 20, 21, 28
arthrocentesis 100–2
    correct placement 101
    hyaluronans 101–2
    synovial fluid removal 101
arthrodesis 110–11
    carpometacarpal thumb joint 111
    first metaatasaphalangeal joint 107
arthropathy, crystal 5, 6, 100
arthroplasty 104–8
    Charnley type low friction 105
    cost-effectiveness analysis 123
    hip 104, 105–6, 107–8
    infected arthroplasty 110

knee 104, 106, 107–8, 109
    life expectancy 107, *108*
    metatarsophalangeal joint 107
    revision operations 108
    shoulder 107
    Stanmore 105–6
    success rate 107
arthroscopy 98, 99, 100, 102
    knee joint 44
aspirin in combination analgesics 88
assessment of OA 55
    elements 55
    functional 56–7
    hand 59–64
    validated instruments 58, **59**
athletes, knee joints 43
audit 76
avascular necrosis 9, 10

β-blockers 92
back pain examination 52
baths 71
behavioural changes 2, 69–71
    in community 72–3
Beighton score 41, 129
bending activities 68
benefits 72–3
benzoxazocines 89
biochemical markers 69
blood, post-traumatic effusion 100
bone
    cysts 12, *13*, 57, 59
    pain 24
    sclerosis 13, 57, 58, 59
bony destruction 5
Bouchard's nodes 5, 7, 59, 60, *61*, 63
    deformed hands 63
bunion *51*
bursitis 24
    anserine 25
    trochanteric 26, 45, 46

caffeine in compound analgesics 88
camphor 86
cancer pain 21
capsaicin **85**, 87
capsicum 86
capsule thickening 14
capsulitis *49*
care
    chronic 120
    expenditure 121
    postoperative 113
    secondary 122

carpometacarpal joint
  arthrodesis 111
  splint 80, *82*
  squaring 61–2, 63
  steroid injection 62
carrying activities 68
cartilage
  breakdown 8, 11
  loss 58
  preserving 102–4
  protection from degradation 1
  proteoglycan matrix 11
  regeneration 11–12
  restoring 102–4
celecoxib 93
Charnley type low friction arthroplasty 105
chiropractic techniques 119
chondrocytes, activity 11
chondroitin 77
chondroitin sulphate 69
chronic care 120
classification of OA 4–5, 55
classification of hand OA 59–65
clavicular joints 48, *49, 50*
climate 8
clinical features of OA 13–16
clinical governance 75–6
clinical pattern 5, 6
  knee OA 21–2
clinical signs 2, 19–21
  suspicious 20–1
co-codamol 88
codeine, paracetamol combination 88
colchicine in gout therapy 27
collagen type 2 genetic abnormality 9
collateral ligaments 42, 99
  integrity test 43
  strains/tears 24
comorbidity 31
complementary therapies 118–19
  costs 122
congenital dislocation of the hip 9, 10
coproxamol 88
cost-effectiveness analysis of arthroplasty 123
costs of OA 121–2
counselling, patient education 66
COX 2 inhibitors 91, 125
  selective/specific 93
coxibs 93
crepitus 15, 21, 30–1, 36
cross fluctuation test 40–1
cruciate ligament 99
  anterior 42
  posterior 42, 43
  repair 99
crystal arthropathy 5, 6, 100
cyclo-oxygenase (COX) 90
  see also COX 2 inhibitors
cyclosporin 92
cytokines 96

day centres 72
debridement and washout 99, 118
debris
  deposition 12
  removal 39

deep vein thrombosis 107
definition of OA 56
Depo-Medrone 95
depression 29, 30, 31
  aerobic exercise 70
  treatment 89
dextropropoxyphene, paracetamol combination 88
diacerain 96
diagnosis 2, 19, 60
  ACR criteria 52, **53**
  alternative 24–9
  referral to secondary care 117
diagnostic triage, back pain 52
diathermy, microwave/short wave 79
diet 70, 76–7
dietary factors 69
digoxin 92
dihydrocodeine 88
  compound analgesics 88
disability
  decrease 124
  fear 30, 31, 66
  prevention in primary care 124
distal interphalangeal joints 60
  erosions 64
  gout 27
  Heberden's nodes 21
  squaring 62
diuretics 92
doctors
  education 69
  visit costs 122
  see also general practitioners
doxycycline 96
draw test, anterior/posterior 42
Dupuytren's contractures 62
dysplasia 10

economics 3
  medical/non-medical approaches 124
education 66–9
  doctors 69
  patient 66–8
  physiotherapy 78
  self-management programmes 124
effusion 5, 16, 22, 98, 99
  aspiration 100
  knee joint 44
  minimal 101
  synovial 100–1
embrocations 86
employment impact 125–6
end-stage disease 17
environmental changes 69–71
  in community 72–3
erythrocyte sedimentation rate (ESR) 28
  polymyalgia rheumatica 28
etodolac 93
exercise 52, 66, 70, 76, 77
  pain 77
  postoperative 112, 113
  quadriceps 79
  warm-up 68
exercise machines 71
expenditure on medical care services 121

facet joints 52
fat pads, knee joint 41
femoral epiphysis, slipped 9, 10, 22
fibromyalgia, differential diagnosis 26
fingers
    stiff/thick 62
    see also grip; hand
fitness, aerobic 70
flexion deformity 34
    fixed 34, 38, 41, 48, 58
flexor sheath, steroid injection 62
footwear 51, 83–4
functional impairment 56–7

gait 34, 35, 36
    antalgic 34, 36, 45
GALS screening examination 127
gate theory of pain 80
gelling 14, 22, 30
gene transfer 96
General Chiropractic Council 119
General Osteopathic Council 119
general practitioners
    barriers to consultation 73–4
    costs of visits 122
    treatment rate 126
genetic susceptibility 5, 7–9
genu recurvatum 41
glucosamine 69, 77
glycosaminoglycan 12
gout 27
    acute 20, 51
    differential diagnosis 24
grating, knee joint 39, 44
grip 38
    impaired 62, 63
gross national product (GNP) 121

haemarthrosis 100
haemochromatosis 9
hallux rigidus 51
hallux valgus 51
hand
    anatomy 60
    assessment 59–64
    deformed 63–4
    obesity 8
    pain 62, 63
    X-rays 64
healthcare
    access to facilities 72
    developments 75
Heberden's nodes 5, 7, 27, 59, 60, 61, 64
    deformed hands 63
    distal interphalangeal joints 21
    gout 27
    hot 59
Helicobacter pylori 125
herbal medicine 119
hip arthroplasty 104, 105–6
    complications 107–8
    total 74
hip joint 5, 6
    childhood problems 9, 10
    dysplasia 10
    examination 34, 35, 36, 44–6, 47, 48
        pain location 44, 45

fixed flexion deformity 48
flexion 34, 35, 46
    occupational hazards 10–11
    osteotomy 108
    pain 24, 26
    rotation 38, 46, 47, 48
        external 46, 47
        internal 46, 47, 48
Hippocratic Oath 119
HLA-A1 B8 gene 76
hobbies 71
holistic approach 119
home equipment 71
home helps 73
homeopathy 119
hormone levels, obesity 8
hormone replacement therapy (HRT) 8, 76
hospital outpatients 116
house, adaptations 71
hyaluronans 12
    arthrocentesis 101–2
    intra-articular 85, 95–6
hyaluronic acid 95, 96
hydantoins 92
Hydrocortisab 95
hydrocortisone acetate 95
hydrotherapy 80
hydroxyapatite crystals deposition 12
hydroxychloroquine 63
Hylan GF20 95
hylans 101
hypermobility, joint 9, 10
    classic signs 129
    knee 41
hyperostosis 50
hypnotherapy 119

ibuprofen 85, 88, 92
illness impact on individual 121–2
infection, excluded 101
infection, haematogenous spread 107
infection rates 107, 113
infection, steroids and systemic signs of
    20–1
inflammation
    flares 89, 93, 94, 101
    knee joint capsule 41
inflammatory response 12
information
    booklets/videos 67, 68
    sources 69
inheritance 76
injection therapy 2, 85, 93–5
injections, compometalcarpal joint 62, 63
injections, flexor sheath 62
injections, metacarpal joint 64
interleukin 1 (IL-1) 96
internet, information for patients 67
interphalangeal joints, squaring 62

joint
    affected 19, 20
    damage 57–8
    destruction 16
    examination 33
        detailed 33–4
        feel 36

knee 38–44
  movement 36, 38
failure 4
functional impairment 15
gelling 30
inflammatory response 12
margins and bony changes 15
movement 36, 38
observation 33–4
pathology 10
protection 66, 70–1
  devices 68
remodelling 11
space
  deposition of debris 12
  narrowing 58
  total loss of 57, 59
square 34
squaring 15
stiffness 14, 22, 30, 62
stress 68
swollen 20
washout 118
X-rays 57, 58, 59, 64
see also crepitus; effusion; hypermobility,
    joint; pain; surgery/surgical
    procedures

knee arthroplasty 44, 102–4, 106–8, 109,
    124
  complications 107–8
  QALY costs 122–3
  total 74, 106
  unicompartmental 110
knee brace 80, 82
knee joint 5
  clinical pattern of OA 21–2
  debris removal 39
  effusions 39–41, 44, 99–100
  examination 36, 38–44
    check list 44
  flexion 38
  grating 39, 44
  hypermobility 41
  inflammation of joint capsule 41
  injury 68
  insecurity 30
  joint line 38
    tenderness 44
  locking 39, 44
  mechanical derangement 39
  movement assessment 41, 42
  MRI 44
  NSAIDs 89–90
  obesity 8
  occupational hazards 10
  osteotomy 108–10
  pain 23, 25
    anterior 39
  patellar taping 80, 81
  periarticular pain 38
  stability 41–2
  synovitis 41
  weight-bearing X-ray 58
  see also collateral ligament; quadriceps
      muscle
knuckles, painful 63

Lederspan 95
leg length, unequal 9, 10
leisure activities 71
Lequesne index for hip and knee 58, 128
lifestyle changes 67, 70–1
ligaments
  injuries 24, 26
  sprains/strains 41
  see also collateral ligaments; cruciate
      ligament
lithium, NSAID interactions 92
loading, abnormal 10–11
locking, knee joint 39
locomotor system, disability 4

magnetic resonance imaging (MRI) 69
  knee joint 44
management 2, 3, 75–6
  education 66–9
  long-term 115–16
  referral to secondary care 117–18
matrix metalloprotease (MMP) activity
    inhibition 96
mechanical interventions 2
mechanical loading, obesity 8
medical approaches, economics 124
medical care services, expenditure 121
meloxicam 93
meniscal cyst 39
meniscal injury 38–9, 43–4
  OA development 98–9
  synovial effusion 100
meniscectomy 98–9
  partial 99
menthol 86
meptazinol 89
metacarpophalangeal joints 62, 63
metatarsophalangeal joint 50–1
  arthroplasties 107
methotrexate 92
methylprednisolone acetate 95
metoclopramide, paracetamol interaction
    86
Milwaukee shoulder 5, 6
minocycline 96
misoprostol 93
mobility
  lack 31
  weight loss 70
mobilization
  back pain 52
  early 111
movement
  joints 36, 38
  knee joint assessment 41, 42
muscles
  pain 24
  strength 70
  weakness 30, 38, 43
  see also abductor muscles; quadriceps
      muscle

nabumetone 93
nefopam 89
nicotinates 86
nitric oxide 96
nitrosated compounds 125

non-medical approaches, economics 124
non-steroidal anti-inflammatory drugs
    (NSAIDs) 1, 2, 88, 89–93
    classical 90, 91
    contraindications 92
    economic assessment 124, 125
    effectiveness 124, 125
    gastrointestinal side-effects 91, **91**, 93
    gout 27
    ineffective 116
    interactions 92
    knee OA 89–90
    limitations to use 91
    misoprostol co-prescription 93
    mode of action 90–1
    pseudogout 28
    side-effects 91, **91**
    symptom control 89
    topical **85**, 86–7
nutritional status 10
nutritional supplements 69
nutritional therapies 119

obesity 8, 68, 76
    arthroplasties 104
occupational hazards 10–11
occupational therapists 81–2
occupational therapy 117
ochronosis 9
oestrogen, menopausal loss 8–9
oestrogen receptors on osteoblasts 8
opiates 116
    compound 88
oral hypoglycaemics, NSAID interactions
    92
osteoblasts, oestrogen receptors 9
osteopathy 119
osteophytes 11, *13*, 15
    marginal 34
osteoporosis 9
osteotomy 107, 108–10, 118
    beneficial effects 109
    exclusion criteria 109–10
    hip joint 108
    knee joint 108–10
    patient selection 109
outcome, patient-centred 123
Oxford Pain Site 88

pacing activities 78
pain 12–13, *14*, 17, 21
    awaiting surgery 116
    bone 24
    definition 56
    diagnostic element 55
    difficulties with everyday activities
        115
    exercise 77
    features 22–3
    gate theory 80
    hand 62, 63
    hip 24, 26
    joint 21, **25**
    knee 23, **25**
        anterior 25, 39
    management 66, 67
        strategies 115

metacarpophalangeal joints 62
muscles 24
periarticular 24, **25**, 26, 36, *37*, *38*
postoperative relief 112
psychological effects 29
reassessment 116
referred 24, **25**, 44
severity 56
site 23–4
subjective 115
treatment strategy changing 116
paracetamol 66, 85–6, 88
    codeine combination 88
    dextropropoxyphene combination 88
patella
    cross fluctuation test 40–1
    resurfacing 106
    tap test 40
patellar taping 80, *81*
patellofemoral OA 39, 71
pathophysiology of OA 1, 11–12
Patient Charter 124
patient-centred outcomes 123
patients
    aids 82–3, *84*
    attitude changing 78
    education 66–8
    expectations 124
    pathways 74, *75*
    postoperative care 111–13
    pressure for referral 118
    primary care choices 123–4
pattern recognition 19
peer review 75–6
pelvic tilt 36
Perthes' disease 9, 10, 22
pharmacological therapy 2, 85
    audit 76
    costs 122
    topical preparations **85**, 86–7
physiotherapy 2, 78–80, *81*, 117
    economic assessment 124
    education 78
    thermal treatments 79
polymyalgia, differential diagnosis 19
polymyalgia rheumatica 29
popliteal cysts 41
prevention
    primary 68
    secondary 68–9
    strategies 68
    tertiary 68, 69
primary care
    disability prevention 124
    patient choices 123–4
    team 75, 116
prognosis 17
proteoglycan matrix 11
proton pump inhibitors 93
proximal interphalangeal joints 60
    gout 27
pseudogout 28
    valgus deformity 36
psychological effects of pain 29
public buildings, access 72
public transport 72
pyrophosphate crystal 28

quadriceps muscle
  exercise 79
  protection of knee 99
  wasting 34, 44
quality adjusted life years (QALY) 123
quality of life 122–3
quinolone antibiotics 92

radiographic techniques 69
radiological changes 4, **55**
'Red Flags' 19–20, **31**, 33, 34
  back pain 52
referral 74, 75
  patient pressure 118
  postoperative for primary care
     111–13
  secondary care 117–18
  surgery 102–4, 118
  within community 116, *117*
rehabilitation, postoperative 111
remodelling, joint 11
research issues 125
rheumatoid arthritis
  differential diagnosis 28–9, 50, 63–4
  valgus deformity 16, 36
risk factors
  general **5**
  genetic 5
  modifiable 68
  obesity 8
  specific **7**, 10–11
rofecoxib 93
rubs 86

Salazopyrin 63
salicylates 86
scarf test *49*, 50
secondary care, costs 122
selective serotonin reuptake inhibitors (SSRIs)
  89
self-help groups 73, 119
  see also support groups
self-management 52
  advice 68
  educational programmes 125
  programmes 120
self-treatment **125**
sensory therapies 119
severe OA 5, 6
sex, prevalence of OA 8–9
shoulder 5, 6
  arthroplasties 107
  movement 38
  septic 20, *21*
showers 71
signs 22–4, **25**
social isolation 31
social services 72–3, 116
social support 116
soft tissue swelling 16
spine 52
spleen 9 line 36
splinting 80, *82*
sports hazards 11
squaring 15, 34
  carpometacarpal joint 61–2, 63
  distal interphalangeal joints 62

interphalangeal joints 62
metacarpophalangeal joints 62
stair lift 71
Stanmore arthroplasties 105–6
sternoclavicular joint 50
steroid injections 20–1, **85**, 93–5
  carpometacarpal joint 62
  contraindications 94
  dosages **95**
  flexor sheath 62
  intra-articular **85**, 93–5
  preparations 95
  side-effects 94
  thumb base 64
steroids
  oral 20–1
  polymyalgia rheumatica 28
stiffness 14
  fingers 62
  morning 30
  see also gelling
stress, joint 68
stretching 68
substance P 87
support groups 68, 116
  see also self-help groups
surgery/surgical procedures 2–3, 104–11
  options 98
  postoperative management 111–13
  referral 102–4, 118
  replacement 74
    total 1, 118
  research 125
  see also arthrodesis; arthroplasty; hip
    arthroplasty; knee arthroplasty;
    osteotomy
swimming 77
symptoms, general 31
synovectomy, medical/surgical 100
synovial effusion 100
  drainage 100–1
synovial fluid, pathophysiology of OA 12
synovitis 16
  crystal-related 93
  knee joint 41
systemic causes 9

taping 80, *81*
tetracycline 96
thermal treatments 79
thiazides, gout control 27
Thomas' test 34, *35*, 48
thumb
  painful 63
  splint 80, *82*
tibiofemoral joint 42
topical preparations 86
topical treatment 2
training, graduated 68
tramadol 89
transcutaneous electrical nerve stimulation
  (TENS) 80
trauma 10
  joint pain 21
  sternoclavicular joint subluxation
    50
Trendelenburg test 34, *35*

triamcinolone hexacetonide 95
tricyclic antidepressants **85**, 89
trochanteric bursa 45, *46*
   see also bursitis, trochanteric
tumour necrosis factor (TNF) 96

ulnar deviation/drift 63
ultrasound, therapeutic 79
uric acid 27

valgus deformity *16*
  correction 84
  pseudogout 28, 36
  rheumatoid arthritis 36
varus angulation/deformity *16, 34, 36*
  correction 84
vitamin C 10
vitamin D 10, 69

warfarin 86
wedge, shoe 83–4
weight loss 66, 70, 76
welfare benefits 72–3
well-being 122, 124
Western Ontario and MacMaster Universities
     Osteoarthritis Index (WOMAC) 58, **59**,
     128
  referral assessment 104
women, elderly 41
work-related problems 122, 125–6
wrist joints 63

X-rays
  hand 64
  joint 57, 58

yttrium, medical synovectomy 100